7·95

REI

108 Questions and Answers

Other titles by Paula Horan

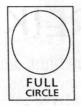

FULL
CIRCLE

Other titles by **Paula Horan**
from FULL CIRCLE

◆ Core Empowerment

◆ An Introduction to Reiki
A 90-minute Video Cassette

REIKI

108 Questions and Answers

Your Dependable Guide
For A Lifetime Of Reiki Practice

PAULA HORAN

Samaya Foundation

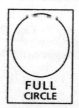

FULL
CIRCLE

REIKI — 108 QUESTIONS AND ANSWERS
© All Rights Reserved, Samaya Foundation, 1998

This Edition, 2001
ISBN 81-7621-034-X

Published by FULL CIRCLE
18-19, Dilshad Garden
G.T., Road Delhi-110 095
Tel : 229 7792   *Fax : 228 2332*

Designing, Typesetting   SCANSET
& Print Production :
18-19, Dilshad Garden, G.T., Road Delhi-110 095
Tel : 228 2467, 229 7792   Fax : 228 2332

Printed at Nu-Tech Photolithographers, Delhi-110 095

PRINTED IN INDIA

Dedicated to my students
in many different parts
of the world,
some of whom
have been my greatest teachers.

Contents

The Five Principles

All About Healing With Reiki

Second Degree Basics

Third Degree Basics

Appendix

Acknowledgments

Thank you, Papaji, for the gift of boundless love and life, without separation.

Thank you, Kate, for making me a Reiki master.

Thank you, all of my students in the four corners of the world, for sharing the incredible presence of Universal Life Force Energy with me.

Thank you, Narayan, for your shoulder to lean on and your knowledge, love and wisdom which I constantly draw on.

Thank you, Shekhar and Poonam for friendship and encouragment.

Thank you, Narendra, Namarata, Nupur, Suresh, Shyam, Nazir, Ranji, Prama, Joginder, Surinder, Rommel, Bruno, George, Renita, Prabha, Brinder, and so many others who have helped me, for your untiring support.

Thank you Lama Drugpa Yeshe Thrinley Odzer for opening the door to some of the innumerable applications of *Men Chhos Rei Kei* — a vast healing mandala of infinite potential.

Thank you, universe, for your innumerable acts of generosity and synchronicity.

Introduction

Have you ever noticed, how occasionally in life, when you plan a new project and begin focusing your energies to get it off the ground, that something else which still needs to be completed, inevitably draws your attention before you can move on to your new project? When you then take up the challenge and follow what is spontaneously arising, you actually clear the way for what you wanted to do in the first place. This is exactly, how *Reiki— 108 Questions And Answers* came about.

Originally, I had planned to write another book at this time, called *True Reiki True Self.* I had even completed the first few chapters, when I had to interrupt the process to go on yet another long extended teaching tour. *True Reiki True Self,* as I envisioned it, would become an inspiring testimony to the unfathomable healing essence of Universal Life Force Energy. It would incorporate some of the history of Dr. Usui from his own journals, which have just come to light, and a discussion of the Tantra from which Reiki is derived. Drawing on my own experience and sharing many of my own stories, I wanted to give the reader a taste of how truly limitless Reiki can be. At least, that was my plan, which will now come to fruition a little later than anticipated.

During my tour, Shekhar and Poonam Malhotra, my publishers in New Delhi, put in a strong request that I first write a book with the bare essentials of Reiki in order to clarify some widespread misunderstandings. Initially, I resisted this project of a "back to basics" Reiki book. Having previously authored three books on Reiki, *Core Empowerment* (1998), *Empowerment Through Reiki* (1989), now available in fifteen languages, and *Abundance Through Reiki* (1995), I felt I had already fully covered the basics. What my publisher and my husband so aptly pointed out, is how profoundly my teaching has changed over the years. It has become simpler and more straightforward. Perhaps, I could convey this to a larger audience.

After getting over my initial resistance, this book developed its own flow and simply happened. It truly wrote itself, and

I derived a lot of pleasure from participating in its creation. The result is a joyful dialogue on the utter beauty, the utter simplicity that is Reiki.

There has been an amazing array of information put out on Reiki in the last few years. Although several good books have been written by a few of the more mature practitioners, the sheer volume of the information now available is sometimes confusing and contradictory to the reader, and is often even totally unrelated to Reiki. Typically, rules from other healing methods are added to Reiki, which aid in the confusion.

For most people in the early stages of Reiki practice, it is hard to grasp just how simple Reiki is. There is a tendency for the beginning practitioner's (and the beginning teacher's) mind to try and make it more complex. The mind (ego) seems to need a lot of unnecessary rules, regulations and accouterments to convince itself that something as simple as Reiki actually works without added on "doo- dads", even though his or her hands palpably tell him or her just the opposite!

In this book, I hope to help a broader public by dispelling a lot of the dis-information that I have been confronted with in my own Reiki classes and which I have heard all too often from other teachers in recent years. Most important, my intention is to explore the basic facets in a clear and simple manner, from my viewpoint, after fourteen years of experience both practicing and teaching Reiki in several different countries.

The information has been kept short and to the point. However, oversimplification has also been carefully avoided. The intention is to present something similar to a reference work, yet in an easy user friendly format. The idea is to provide you with something like a companion or guide that can address the queries which inevitably surface.

When formulating the questions, I was able to draw on

the many classes that I have taught since 1987. I purposely chose the questions that my students most often ask me during or directly after a Reiki class.

Teaching happens in a natural flow when it takes the form of a dialogue. The question and answer format seemed appropriate in order to recreate the sense of engaging in a dialogue with the reader. The philosophers of ancient Greece did not hold professorships. They went about Athens and talked to just about everyone. Likewise, the Buddha didn't sit under a tree to scribble scriptures on palm leaves. Instead, he wandered all over Northern India and engaged people in conversations whenever they were interested in listening to what he had to share.

When I teach a class, people ask me questions and I respond spontaneously to whatever is invoked by the questioner. This is precisely the feeling I tried to achieve in *Reiki — 108 Questions and Answers*, the feeling of a live dialogue between student and teacher. Here, many of the topics are dealt with which regularly come up during a Reiki class. You could say, the book is the next best thing to taking a class with me. The only drawback, is that I am not personally present to clarify points or dispel doubts. However, if you use this book as intended, you will find that a careful examination of the pertinent passages will eventually give you the answers that you were looking for, which are actually already inside of you. In order to ask a question, you already have to have intuitively grasped a large part of the answer. Answers are really just to dispel doubts.

This is why the book is also called *Your Dependable Guide For A Lifetime Of Reiki Practice*. Whenever you are in doubt or feel that a certain question about the basic practice of Reiki has been left unanswered, go back and look up the relevant sections of the text.

Let's face it. Humans are forgetful. Even if you pay close attention, you are bound to disregard a lot of things that were mentioned in your Reiki class. Furthermore, studies have shown that even good students on the average absorb only 35% of the information given to them at any one time. Which explains why you have to go back and study the things which you really want to learn. Since the human mind generally doesn't have the capacity to absorb all of the information which it receives, it helps to have a reliable source you can go back to whenever you need clarification.

This book fulfills yet another need. Considering the previously mentioned fact that usually only 35% of the information given at any one time is retained, what do you think will happen to basic Reiki knowledge, which can only be integrated experientially, if passed on through a line of teachers who became Reiki masters within a week or a month, and then proceeded to initiate others into mastership shortly thereafter? How much accurate knowledge will remain after three or four generations of teachers and students of this kind? Under such conditions, a book of basic Reiki questions and answers can be of great assistance for those who want to go back to its real roots.

Overall, I have kept the book within the boundaries of Reiki, as taught by Hawayo Takata. Some short references are made, however, to other authentic transmissions of Universal Life Force Energy, also going back to Dr. Usui, the founder of modern day Reiki. My source for these little tidbits of information was Lama Drugpa Yeshe Thrinley Odzer who intitiated me into Men Chhos Rei Kei, a complete system of advanced healing practices. It is derived from the writings of Dr. Usui found in his commentaries and diaries as well as from the *Tantra Of The Lightening Flash Which Heals The Body And Illumines The Mind*, a Shingon Buddhist scripture and the source of inspiration for Dr. Usui's own realization. As these teachings are meant to be revealed in a direct student/teacher interaction I have only included material that pertains to the history of Reiki, and is therefore of general interest.

In any event, at present, most Reiki practitione.s can trace their lineage back to Dr. Usui and the Usui Method Of Natural Healing (*Usui Shiki Ryoho*) through Mrs. Takata and one of her twenty-two master students who made Reiki popular all around the world. Therefore, particular emphasis has been put on her form of Reiki, simply because it is the most widely practiced, and yet often the most misunderstood, even to the point of complete distortion. *108 Questions And Answers* is my own contribution to help clear some of the most common misunderstandings in a gentle and non-judgmental manner.

That there are altogether 108 questions and answers listed in this book is of course, no mere coincidence. The total of the digits in 108 is 9. Nine, in turn is the only number which reproduces itself as the sum of the digits when multiplied by any integer number. For example: *3x9=27 and 2+7=9. Or: 4x9=36 and 3+6=9;* and so forth. Therefore, 9 is seen as the number of completion. As the product of 9x12, 108 is regarded as a particularly auspicious number, which is why it was chosen for this book to convey the auspicious presence of Universal Life Force Energy.

For further information, in the appendix, I have included an essay on the full body treatment, its effect on the endocrine system, the systems' connection to the immune system, and its role in healing because this is where Mrs. Takata focused her attention in her own treatments, besides treating the major organs of the body.

In most other books on Reiki, references to the endocrine system remain scanty. Instead, their focus is on more esoteric and etheric levels of organization. For this basic presentation of the principles of hands on and distant healing with Universal Life Force Energy, I have refrained from getting too esoteric. In this instance, it did indeed seem counterproductive.

In a second essay, I have discussed at length the reason why Reiki may prove particularly helpful in this day and age, as each individual's very own personal declaration of independence from drugs and unnecessary outside interventions.

Through the actual practice of Reiki, all of the answers you will ever need will come to you as if by osmosis. It is important to remember that all "in"-formation comes from the outside and is ultimately mind-stuff. Therefore, it is essential not to get stuck in or attached to any of the answers contained in the text. It is better to let the answers instead act as an inspiration to help you create your own response — to help you get in touch with your own inner knowing.

Practicing Reiki supports you in tapping your own feelings. All of *your* answers lie within the superior intelligence of your heart. Thus, the ability to feel, which Reiki promotes due to its very essence as heart energy, will help you to find your own answers. For those who need support in letting go of resistance to feelings, this book may provide insights to assist you further along the path.

Ultimately, the proof in the pudding regarding Reiki is in the practice. I wish you much comfort, ease and joy in your work with Reiki. Share it with yourself and others as often as possible, because the more you call on Universal Life Force Energy the quicker it will respond.

BASIC REIKI

What is Reiki ?

Most commonly, the word Reiki refers to a simple hands-on healing technique, a form of energy medicine which was rediscovered by Dr. Mikao Usui in Japan in the late 19th century. Dr. Usui chose the term Reiki to describe Universal Life Force Energy which calms the mind and raises a person's life force. Through the use of soothing hands laid on the body in certain positions, the process of healing is accelerated. The essence of this form of healing is passed on from teacher to student through a series of mystic initiations which in Reiki, like in the Tantric forms of Buddhism in Japan or Tibet, are called attunements or empowerments.

In actuality, Reiki is the fundamental nature or substratum of the universe, and the *Usui Method Of Natural Healing* is an easy way of giving back to yourself more of what you already fundamentally are: Universal Life Force Energy. You literally recharge yourself with that, which at the deepest level, you have always been.

In quantum physics as well as hermetic science, energy is recognized as the fundamental nature of existence. In truth there is no solid matter. Thus, the human body, its thoughts and emotions are all composed of energy oscillating at various frequencies. The denser the vibration, the more apt we are to experience discomfort or dis-ease. The freer the vibration, the greater the chance for natural health, abundance, beauty, satisfaction and well-being.

Through getting the body/mind in touch with Universal Life Force Energy, its very own substratum, Reiki can release the individual in a gentle and gradual manner from age old restrictions and bondage, and allow over time to first experience vibrant health and balance, and finally experience freedom and unity.

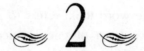

Where does Reiki come from?

In its outer appearance as energy medicine, Reiki has its real roots in India, having passed through Tibet and China to Japan, where it was rediscovered by Dr. Usui. In its unlimited inner potential, Reiki comes from nowhere in particular because it is everywhere and exists as everything. In this aspect of Universal Life Force Energy, Reiki is unknowable and ungraspable, and yet can be directly experienced by everyone at every moment due to its all-pervasive nature.

As the *Usui Method Of Natural Healing*, Reiki is but one branch of the many different healing arts whose origins go back into prehistoric times. Specifically, Reiki belongs to the medical traditions which originated in South, Central and East Asia. According to Dr. Usui's own writings, Reiki as we have known it so far in the West, is a synthesis of a seven level

Tantric teaching developed for lay people of any religious or philosophical persuasion, and is closely connected with the scriptural and energy transmissions or empowerments related to the Healing Buddha.

In a deeper sense, as Universal Life Force Energy itself, Reiki is the substratum or underlying nature of everything. It exists everywhere. Due to our identification with the body and its five senses we have forgotten that, in actuality, we are the very unlimitedness of being itself. We don't recall the powers granted to us: that by simply being open and aware, we can draw whatever resources we need directly to us (much like Christ manifesting the fish and the loaves, or Sai Baba manifesting *vibhuti*).

Through the attunements or empowerments of Reiki (which re-establish the direct energetic channel .we have for Universal Life Force Energy to flow through), we begin to reconnect (or simply notice) the direct link we've always had with all the energy there is. We begin to draw in directly what we need from what at first seems to come from the outside, and slowly regain the knowledge that all we are is within Heart (including our bodies).

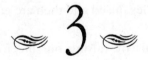

How does Reiki heal?

By calming the mind and raising the life force energy in the body.

The body is actually energy vibrating at a certain frequency, and all its frequencies have their own natural flow.

However, when we make a judgment about something (rather than discernment), the judgment gets stored in the cellular structure of the body in the form of a physical and/or emotional block. Emotions are a reaction to our thoughts or judgments about people and life's situations. Since they distort the natural frequencies, negative thoughts or judgments are experienced as dense or uncomfortable vibrations. Such thoughts may turn into headaches, tension, stomach aches or ulcers. Rage and anger or grief held in the body can easily turn into tumors. In the same way, mental control "trips" or the power trips we bought into from others can turn into rheumatoid arthritis.

Provided we stick to the tried and proven procedures outlined by any good, traditional Reiki teacher, Reiki, over time, may actually heal all of these blockages. Reiki exposes them to the much higher vibratory frequency of Universal Life Force Energy which can then penetrate and dissolve any block.

By simple laying on of hands over the entire body so that it can draw the energy it needs, Reiki helps us to feel our feelings fully so they can easily pass through the body/mind and not get stuck. Old stuck thoughts (through treatment) have their frequencies raised and then are enabled to also pass through.

Thus Reiki heals by raising our life force frequency.

≈ 4 ≈

Who is Dr. Mikao Usui ?

Dr. Mikao Usui is the founder of the modern day Reiki movement. According to recently found information, he was a Shingon Buddhist priest, family man and physician, and the son of the secretary of the mayor of Tokyo during the late Meiji era. Born in the latter half of the 19th century, he died in the mid twenties of this century. Dr. Usui was of minor aristocracy and as a young man was originally encouraged to go into business, but as this was not his true proclivity, he instead studied the Japanese and Chinese healing arts, and later Western allopathic medicine with Christian missionary doctors.

Due to a powerful spiritual experience in his late twenties during a serious bout with cholera, Usui felt drawn to the spiritual side of life. A true Bodhisattva, he rediscovered a very ancient healing art revealed in a 1100 year old Buddhist manuscript: *The Tantra Of The Lightening Flash That Heals The Body And Illumines The Mind* which included a few practices that he adopted for the benefit of lay people of any religion or background.

Dr. Usui created a brief synthesis of the essence of this seven level Tantric teaching as Reiki (Universal Life Force Energy), as it conveys the healing energy through the simple laying on of soothing hands. He divided this first level of the teaching into Three Degrees and shared his knowledge and experience in his own medical practice with many people. The more subtle aspects, however, were only taught to his nineteen close students, the foremost among them being Dr. Watanabe in the full system of all seven levels, and Dr. Hayashi in the system of the synthesis, called Reiki.

5

How is Reiki different from other healing methods?

Reiki is a form of energy medicine similar to *Touch For Health* or *Pranic Healing*. The essential difference is Reiki's utter simplicity (besides a few hand positions, there is no methodology to learn) and the recognition that no one ever heals anyone else: that all healing is pure Grace and just *happens*.

For example, if I lay my hands on you to "do" a treatment, your body will simply draw what it needs through the channel. You can actually be doubtful or skeptical, because Reiki ultimately transcends the mind; however, you do need to be at least open to the possibility of receiving Reiki. Your body will then of its own innate intelligence simply draw in what it needs.

Thus in Reiki, I don't have to sit there and try to make the energy flow. Simply by my intention to share a treatment, the energy begins to be *drawn* into the other, and this is the key: Reiki is always drawn, never sent, even at the Second Degree level, when distant treatments are shared.

Thus, one only has to learn how to listen to one's hands. Through the recognition of our true state of "non-doing" (that everything which happens in the universe happens due to pure Grace), Reiki could be aptly called the simplest of all healing arts.

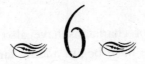

Is there more than one form of authentic Reiki ?

Yes, there are several authentic forms and lineages of Reiki, but not everything that calls itself Reiki actually is Reiki. Among the authentic forms and lineages are the following:

1) *Traditional Reiki* as taught through the direct lineage of Usui, Hayashi, Takata and her twenty-two direct students (provided that every master further down the line has kept the transmission pure and teaches it in its essential form).

2) All lineages that go back to Dr. Usui through Dr. Hayashi and his student Sensei Takeuchi, a Zen monk who received a different set of teachings from Dr. Hayashi than Mrs. Takata.

3) *Men Chhos Rei Kei International*, because it is based on Dr. Usui's own notes and on the *Tantra Of The Lightening Flash Which Heals The Body And Illumines The Mind* and its additional empowerments which were Dr. Usui's own source of inspiration.

4) *Usui Reiki Ryoho Gakkei*, the traditional Reiki which has been practiced in Japan itself in an unbroken lineage and is not connected to Mrs. Takata.

Since Dr. Usui had altogether nineteen close students, there may be other authentic forms and lineages of Reiki that still remain quietly hidden by the wayside.

However, due to the popularity of the *Usui Method Of Natural Healing* and the increasing demand for it around the world, a number of charlatans have also appeared. A few disreputable people have begun adding fantasy symbols and attunements and have created new forms and haphazard healing techniques to which, solely as a marketing ploy, they fraudulently attach the word Reiki. I do not wish to mention any of them specifically but leave that to your own discernment. Usually their fraudulent creations carry as their name a catchy noun or combination of nouns in connection with the word Reiki.

Since the Reiki channel is always inherently there in all sentient beings, a charismatic charlatan can also help you feel some form of energy. If you believe in them, it will work up to a certain point. What you will be missing though, is the connection with the ancient lineage of Reiki as conveyed by a series of self realized beings through the vehicle of the attunements.

Very few Reiki masters or teachers (the word Reiki master is used in a similar context to a master craftsperson) practicing today are self realized. This means that the seed energy for the opening of the Reiki channel is carried only by the attunements, and not in but rather *through* the teacher him- or herself. Thus it is important to at least find someone in one of the proper lineages who can share attunements that go back to Dr. Usui and the ancient lineage of practitioners.

☙ 7 ☙

What are attunements ?

Attunements (or empowerments) are the essential ingredients in any Reiki class. At the First Degree level there are four attunements, and at Second and Third Degree, one attunement respectively.

Reiki attunements are essentially a ritualized ceremony which convey the essence or seed kernel of that which you already are (Universal Life Force Energy), in such a way that the initial veils of ignorance are removed so that you can begin to experience the direct link that you have always had with all the energy there is (because that is what you truly are).

As within any ancient tradition (Reiki is at least two thousand years old) where empowerments are given, such as in the empowerments given by Tibetan Lamas or Shingon Buddhist masters, it is necessary to find a master teacher within that same tradition who has received and integrated the oral teachings and imbibed the wisdom energetically through practice and through a direct connection with a living master in the tradition. Thus it is that Reiki empowerments can be properly given only by a Reiki master/teacher who is in the direct lineage of Dr. Mikao Usui.

Some people now believe that Dr. Usui was a reincarnation of Kukai, the Buddhist monk who brought the original teaching which incorporates what Usui later called Reiki to Japan in the eighth century CE. If this is so, it would thus be no surprise that after much concerted effort, using spiritual practices contained in the teaching, Dr. Usui would then be enabled to receive the empowerments directly. As there were no living masters alive in Japan at his time who remembered the empowerments, Usui had no choice but to perform certain spiritual practices unassisted until his own veils of ignorance fell away.

It is thus through the determination and Grace of Dr. Usui that the empowerments of this ancient teaching were reinstated and carried forth. Empowerments from a self realized being such as Usui carry the "mustard seed" for others to more easily shed the ignorance that keeps us in both mental and physical suffering.

It is my experience, due to the flood of students seeking to be reattuned, that most of the forms of so-called "Reiki" with a lot of superfluous added on names and probably newly invented symbols and abbreviated attunements carry very little essence behind them. Thus it is important to connect with a teacher in one of the direct lineages of Dr. Mikao Usui.

Attunements on a practical level, raise a person's life force energy and reawaken them to the Reiki channel so that they may treat themselves, and as an added benefit also treat others. At the First Degree level, much focus is directed toward the physical body so that at the cellular level the vibratory rate is amplified. People often experience emotional and physical cleansings as a result, as much density is sloughed off.

At the Second Degree level the amplification seems to center more on the etheric or energy body which contains the chakras or main subtle energy centers. Further emotional and physical cleansings can occur with an accompanying opening at an intuitive level. Because of this opening, which sometimes brings psychic abilities with it, many people become excited, and are then drawn to do Third Degree prematurely.

The Third Degree attunement, if given too early, seems not to amplify your energy, but only your ego, whenever you are not properly prepared, as the focus of Third Degree is actually about dropping your power "trip". Thus we see tremendous ignorance today being acted out by many so-called "Reiki masters". Overall, the attunements affect each individual according to their own evolution, and never bring out more than you are ready for. The Third Degree attunement is the one attunement that should be postponed as long as is appropriate, in order to gain full benefit.

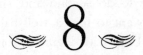

How can I tell if I have chosen a suitable Reiki master?

From the previous question and answer it should now be obvious why discernment is essential in choosing a Reiki teacher. Ideally, you want to choose a Reiki master who carries both the essence (through a detached yet joyful and openhearted noticing and sharing of the ever-presence of Universal Life Force Energy) and can convey the attunements of the Usui Method Of Natural Healing.

Some of the key questions you may want to ask a prospective Reiki teacher are: 1. *How long have you practiced Reiki?* (Hopefully at least three years before becoming a master.) 2. *Can you trace your lineage back to Dr. Usui?* (The attunements which are given should be in Dr. Usui's transmission to ensure that you will receive the essence or seed kernel of Grace which helps to truly unveil the Reiki channel.) 3. *Do you feel at peace in your master's/teacher's presence?* (Although sometimes a true teacher may challenge the status quo — your ego — and temporarily make you feel off balance, overall you should feel a sense of peace in their presence.)

Any other questions which come to mind are pertinent (otherwise they wouldn't come up). Also, notice if they are overly impressed with all the people "they have healed" (Remember, in Reiki, healing just happens!), or maintain a sense of equanimity about themselves and life in general.

A genuine Reiki master will never proselytize Reiki. They most assuredly will be enthusiastic, but especially, should never push people to do Second and Third Degree.

Basically, you want to find a well balanced person with a positive outlook. University degrees, professional certificates or logos on letterheads are not so important as is basic common sense. The final sign for a good teacher is that in an overall sense they challenge you, but at the same time make you feel good about yourself. In other words, they don't blow themselves (their precious ego) up at your expense. They don't make you feel small, but rather inspire you to directly experience that you are THAT, Universal Life Force Itself!

Is there such a thing as a grand master in Reiki?

No, there isn't. Dr. Usui, who through arduous effort rediscovered Reiki and became the founder of the entire modern day Reiki movement, never even thought of referring to himself as "grand master". If he didn't, why should anyone else? In all spiritual traditions the world over, honorary titles are sometimes bestowed upon those rare individuals who totally live what they teach and are surrounded by an aura of absolute realization. In that sense, Dr. Usui and someone like him actually could be considered a true grand master. The point is, that he never called himself such. The bottom line is: whoever finds it necessary to call him- or herself "grand master" is still far removed from true mastership, let alone "grand" mastership.

Another factor that contributed to the creation of literally dozens of "grand masters" can be found in the improper way Third Degree has been taught by splitting it into 3A and 3B. A new terminology was created to decipher the difference between the two. There is no such thing as a "half master" You either are or you aren't. Some inexperienced Reiki masters adopted the idea that giving the Third Degree attunement would help others in their spiritual growth and "boost" their power. Some ill-informed people even teach 3A in a class format and give large numbers the Third Degree attunement as a marketing ploy. Those who later decide they want to teach can then pay another fee and learn how to do the attunements and teach. Because students who had only received the Third Degree symbol and attunement (3A) began to call themselves Reiki masters, some of the people who had completed 3B opted for calling themselves "grand masters" to make themselves stand out.

Nowadays, there are many people calling themselves "grand masters" who don't even have 3A or 3B or any authentic Reiki attunement for that matter. The whole thing has become a joke. A true master (in the sense of having mastered the ego/mind) would never even call himself master, let alone add the title "grand". For myself, I use the title Reiki master much in the same way as a master craftsperson would. In other words, no claim is made beyond the ability to share correct Reiki attunements that go back to Dr. Usui.

✍ 10 ✍

How is Reiki taught?

Reiki is taught in three stages or Degrees in order to help the student properly integrate the empowerments or attunements (it takes 21 days just for the physical body to process the attunements at each level). Teaching Reiki in stages also helps the student to gain adequate experience and understanding of the subtlety of Reiki at each level.

First Degree Reiki can be given over a four day period (one attunement per day), or minimally a two day period, as there needs to be at least 24 hours between the second and third attunement (there are four attunements in First Degree). Two full days or four full evenings are required for the First Degree class in order for the students to properly learn the hand positions and complete enough treatments to gain confidence to work on their own.

First Degree treatments should be practiced a minimum of three months before considering Second Degree. Even a six month or much longer period is a good idea to reap the full benefit of Second Degree. Second Degree can be taught in only 4 or 5 hours, but I have found it beneficial to show my students additional possibilities for using Second Degree, therefore I usually teach for a day and a half, or two full days with a larger group.

First and Second Degree are the practitioner level. They cover every aspect you need to integrate, in order to become proficient in applying this ancient healing art. No further "boost" is needed to empower yourself spiritually. Third Degree is only for people who want to teach Reiki, and should not be considered until a student has completed at least three years of not only self-treatments, but additionally, hundreds of treatments on others, ideally in a clinical practice or similar situation.

Third Degree is not meant to be taught in a seminar or divided into 3A and 3B (there are no "half masters"!). I personally will only train master students after I have known them and worked with them for at least a year, and who have a least three years of experience behind them. The master training is a one to one procedure, and generally takes a full year to complete.

In addition to the three years of experience with Reiki, a Third Degree or master student should ideally have completed some self-assessment work beforehand. My own Third Degree students are required to take the *Core Empowerment Training* at least three times to help quiet the mind and prepare them to become teachers (refer to my book *Core Empowerment: A Course In The Power Of The Heart, With Commentaries For Advanced Reiki Practitioners*, Full Circle, New Delhi, 1998).

I consider the master/student relationship at Third Degree level to be a life time commitment for both parties, and therefore do not take it lightly.

11

How many Degrees of Reiki are there?

Reiki, the *Usui Method Of Natural Healing*, is actually a parallel teaching for lay people of any background of a seven level Tantric teaching. To more easily convey the various attunements of Reiki, Dr. Hayashi divided Reiki into Three Degrees.

The First Degree attunes or aligns the student to the Reiki frequency through four empowerments. This allows the student to experience a direct connection with Universal Life Force Energy so that they can begin to channel the energy to themselves and others. After a period of adjustment and a lot of practice on self and others (minimally three months) Second Degree can be conveyed. One attunement or empowerment is given, and three symbols are taught which enable the energy to transcend time and space.

At the Second Degree level distant treatments can be shared with others, but an emphasis is put on healing personal (emotional and mental) wounds from the past. As old past hurts are healed, a new self-confidence emerges which helps to release protective ego related patterns.

Third Degree is the teaching level of Reiki and should only be considered after a minimum of three years of practice, and this only if there is a strong desire to become a Reiki teacher. The focus of the Third Degree attunement is not so much on amplifying your healing power, as it is on empowering you to convey the attunements. There is one attunement and one symbol learned in the Third Degree training, plus the procedure for the First, Second and Third Degree attunements. Generally Third Degree is taught over a one year period. The student organizes and co-teaches several classes and has regular consultations with the master.

Ideally, at the Third Degree level, the commitment between master and student is for a life long relationship, based on respect and the full awareness that at the deepest level there is neither master nor student but only Universal Love and Life Energy at play with Itself.

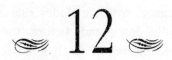

12

Why are there Degrees ?

The Three Degrees essentially correspond to three different combinations of attunements which energetically promote different shifts or openings. Although they are interrelated as one organic whole, the Three Degrees serve different purposes. The first set of altogether four attunements into First Degree is to be given in close succession and then integrated for a period of at least three weeks. To absorb fully what you have learned may take a few months. The one attunement for Second and Third Degree respectively also need time for proper assimilation.

There are several distinct steps in the integration of Reiki. After the four First Degree attunements the body/mind goes through a 21-day cleanse process. A period of self treatment (and preferably a number of treatments on others) is desirable to help the student gain confidence in the treatment process. Although the energy is palpable during the First Degree class, the human mind which is beset with doubt, easily forgets what it has experienced. Thus, consistent daily practice in the first few weeks is needed to gain confidence because for many, simply learning to touch the body and listen to the hands can take some time.

If Reiki treatments are given on a daily basis, the life force energy continues to increase gradually over time, and the next attunement can then be better integrated.

The attunement into Second Degree is much more fully appreciated after an extended practice at the First Degree level. Second Degree, which includes one attunement, also needs to be fully integrated before the Third Degree attunement (if one desires to teach Reiki) can be given.

Basically, the Three Degrees delineate three distinct processes which each need time to be fully assimilated by the individual. Although there are basic guidelines to be followed in terms of time and practice between Degrees, occasionally there may be exceptions to the rule.

Some people actually find it helpful to wait a few years between First and Second Degree in order to allow the practice of Reiki to work to its full benefit. Also they may never even consider Third Degree because they are content to apply Reiki, but have no desire to become Reiki teachers. The point here is that it is important to follow the voice of your heart and not succumb to any outside pressure which tries to convince you that you need Third Degree in order for your Reiki to become more "powerful". This is pure baloney sauce! There are many First and Second Degree practitioners who are more mature in their practice than others who now call themselves Reiki masters.

13

Why is there a fee for Reiki?

In order to help students appreciate such a "pearl of great price", and to ensure that people who take First Degree are actually motivated enough to use it, Mrs. Takata always encouraged an exchange of energy regarding Reiki. It is very similar to going into a doctor's office where you pay a fee for medical advice. If you have paid hard earned money for your advice, you are much more likely to follow it.

After giving many Reiki treatments for quite some time, according to Mrs. Takata, Dr. Usui noticed that many people took the results for granted, and did not really take responsibility for their own health (much like many people who want an instant pill or cure all from a doctor, but who will not correct the bad diet or lack of exercise which caused the problem in the first place). People generally paid the equivalent of doctor's visit for a Reiki treatment (Dr. Usui was after all, a physician with a wife and two children).

To help people learn First Degree Reiki so that they could take better care of themselves, Mrs. Takata accepted or charged the equivalent of a week's worth of labor; for Second Degree the equivalent of month's worth of labor; and for Third Degree the equivalent of a year's worth of labor. After such payment, people were no longer beholden to her and could gain the most benefit.

Today unfortunately, many people have turned Reiki into a business and have no concept of the rationale behind charging for Reiki. Some give it away for practically nothing in order to be "competitive", with the result that the students often don't appreciate what they have received. Others due to their charisma and popularity charge exorbitant fees, yet teach low quality classes where their students are given little or no time to learn how to practice simple and straightforward Reiki.

Over the past fifteen years, there has been much controversy in the Reiki community about the issue of the correct fees. At this point, there is no need to add fuel to the fire because to the intelligent observer the question of the right fee resolves itself. Reiki empowers you to become healthy and whole through applying the very energy you are actually made of. If you take this statement as a fact, you'll ultimately cherish the gift of Reiki and be willing to pay for it. On the other hand, if you don't even have an inkling of the depth and potential of the Reiki energy, then taking a Reiki class is probably not a good idea for you anyway.

Also, nowhere did Dr. Usui himself state that the exchange of energy has to be made in hard cash. You can be creative and think of other forms when they are called for, like a work of art or a piece of jewelry or certain services. However, I would strongly suggest that the teacher not become the banker for the student. The exchange of energy should be completed before the attunements are given to avoid any source for future conflicts.

The bottom line is: whether looking for a class or a treatment, discernment is needed. It is best not to necessarily go with the cheapest offer, but to look for quality in the practitioner or teacher.

FIRST DEGREE BASICS

⇜ 14 ⇝

What is First Degree Reiki?

First Degree helps you to align with Reiki energy so that you can channel it to yourself and others, for the purpose of healing, through the simple laying on of hands. It helps put you in touch with the direct link you've always had (but never realized) with all the energy you'll ever need to heal yourself, by calming the mind and raising your life force energy.

Due to thousands of years of conditioning, that you are not good enough, that you don't know enough, and the belief that all you need is outside of yourself, you've developed an acute sense of separation or subject/object relationship with reality. If you look around, you will see this for yourself. Everything in human society seems to confirm that we are terribly alone and very much lacking in one thing or another. This only amplifies our sense of neediness so that we begin to seek outside of ourselves to fill the vaccum.

Basically every single ad in magazines or on TV reminds you of what you don't (but should) have, whereas in reality, deep down, you *are* unbelievably rich: You are the universe Itself with all its inherent wealth, although not in the ordinary ego sense of these words. We tend to forget that in actual fact all is energy, that even our bodies are a certain vibratory frequency, that indeed everything is vibration, and that there is no solid matter. Thus there are really no separate entities or selves and we are already totally connected to all knowledge.

Who we really are is the ocean of consciousness itself. Each one of us, who seems so separate due to the information our five senses give us, is very much like a "separate" wave in the ocean. There is an appearance of a lot of different waves, but actually, *all the waves are the ocean itself,* and totally inseparable. Each one of us is like a wave who has forgotten who we truly are, and due to this forgetfulness we also don't experience our true nature.

First Degree Reiki helps remove one of the veils of forgetfulness, so that a palpable connection is reinstated with the unlimited energy of the universe. At First Degree level there may still be a sense that Reiki comes from the outside to heal the body and calm the mind. With practice over time, a recognition dawns of a healing of a far greater scope than simple physical ailments. This healing will gradually remove a sense of separation and bring you to a direct experience of unity.

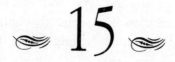

How many attunements are there?

In First Degree Reiki there are four attunements. The focus at this stage is to fine tune the physical vehicle, to actually raise the life force energy at a cellular level, so that the body can receive or channel greater quantities of life force energy to both itself and others. The purpose of the attunements is not to open chakras or awaken the Kundalini, although sometimes certain openings may occur. The focus of First Degree attunements is to reinstate the Reiki channel, the direct link we've always had (but could not perceive due to our conditioning) to the Universal Life Force Energy which we truly are.

The attunements can be given one per day over a four day period or minimally over two days with 24 hours between the second and third attunement. Never should all four attunements be given in one day! If they are, this is a dead give away that you are not receiving the Reiki empowerments as passed down by Dr. Usui.

The first empowerment attunes the heart and thymus on both the physical and the etheric level and establishes the Reiki channel. The second empowerment affects the thyroid gland and on an etheric level helps to open the communication center. It also raises the life force energy of the nervous system which then needs time to adjust. The third attunement affects the pineal gland (which, etherically, corresponds to the third eye) and the hypothalamus which rules the body's mood and temperature. A sense of calm or peacefulness often occurs after this attunement. The fourth empowerment is the final "sealing in" process, and sets the channel in so that you'll never lose it.

All four attunements have an effect on the entire endocrine system, and continue to reap their benefit during the 21-day cleanse process, as much of the dross in the blocked areas is let go off.

Your Reiki channel may "atrophy" over a period of years if you don't use it, but it will always remain with you ready to be reinstated whenever you call upon it, once all four attunements have been completed.

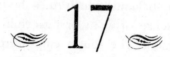

16

How long does it take to learn Reiki?

Taking a Reiki class is not like any class you've ever taken. There is nothing intellectual about First Degree Reiki, so there are no books to read or tests to take. Since it is totally experiential it is very easy and enjoyable to learn (my youngest student was four years old). Within a two day period, most people can assimilate the basic hand positions and begin practicing on others as well as on themselves. After the attunements reestablish your connection with Reiki, it is then a simple process of learning to listen to your hands so that you will know how long to keep them on each position on the body.

17

How often should I practice?

Ideally you can treat yourself every day, morning and evening. I generally give myself a treatment when I lay down in bed at night, starting with the head and throat. I often just make it to my heart and fall asleep. In the morning when I wake up, I start where I left off and continue down the body, then sit up to do my knees, feet and back.

For First Degree students, I also recommend that you treat seven different people three times each for the first 21 days after the class. This helps you gain more confidence in your ability to feel and share Universal Life Force Energy, as you receive feedback from others. Furthermore, as you give Reiki treatments, you also receive a treatment indirectly, for the energy has to flow through you first before being drawn through your hands into the other person and a certain amount, as needed, remains with you. The mind also tends to settle down more quickly with the extra practice and makes your self treatments easier.

～ 18 ～

What are the basics taught in a First Degree class?

After receiving the four attunements of First Degree, you are taught all the hand positions which cover the endocrine glands (which correspond to the major energy centers or chakras) and all the major organs.

Every Reiki teacher shares the background of Reiki with an in-depth history of Dr. Mikao Usui. Most also cover information on his students Dr. Chujiro Hayashi and Hayashi's student Hawayo Takata who brought Reiki to America and Canada, and from there to the entire world. Most Reiki masters today can trace their lineage through Mrs. Takata.

An overview of First, Second and Third Degree is given, and all the essentials (many of which are answered in this book) regarding treatments. The five principles are also discussed, and there is always sufficient time for one or two extended question and answer sessions.

Most of the course however, is devoted to hands on practice: self treatment, group treatments, and giving and receiving at least one full body treatment with a partner.

≈ 19 ≈

What is the structure of a First Degree class?

First Degree is organized in four, four hour segments. Some teachers share the attunements over four successive evenings. Most teachers, however, lead Reiki classes on the weekend for the convenience of their students, usually from 9:00am to 5:00pm, with two morning and two afternoon sessions. The first session usually covers the history and background of Reiki, the hand positions for self treatment, the first two attunements (if the class is given on a weekend) and self treatments. There is usually a lunch break, and the afternoon is a long session of group treatments with a question and answer session.

On the second day (in a two day class) the morning begins with the third and fourth attunements, more group treatments and a discussion of the Reiki principles. After a lunch break each participant has the opportunity to give a full body treatment to a partner and then receive a treatment from the same partner. Generally, there is a group discussion with question and answers at the end of the class.

20

What are the hand positions and how can I treat specific ailments?

Every position on the body is a possible Reiki hand position, so there are no set rules of what can and cannot be treated. Ultimately, Reiki energy will always be drawn where it is most needed in the body so there is no need to worry about putting your hands on a "wrong" position. With this all stated notwithstanding, there are some basic positions on the body which were recommended by Mrs. Takata to be covered in a full body treatment. Her main focus was to treat all the major organs and the endocrine system.

I generally recommend that students either purchase or borrow from a library, a good anatomy picture book, in order to learn the proper placement of the major organs and endocrine glands after I first demonstrate them in the class. Mrs. Takata never discussed treating chakras which has become so popular today (perhaps partially due to my book *Empowerment Through Reiki*, written ten years ago, which was the first to discuss the chakras and their treatment at length), but emphasized the importance of the endocrine glands which control the body's chemistry and happen to be in the same position as the seven main chakras or energy centers.

To begin a treatment I generally start at the head, which helps to immediately calm the mind and release stress. I start by placing my palms over my eyes while simultaneously covering the sinuses and third eye or pineal gland. I next place my hands on the temples, ears, and then occipital lobes at the base of the skull. For the fifth position, I place one hand over both occipital lobes and the other over the forehead. This position releases headaches, stress and tension. The next position is one hand over the throat and one hand behind the back of the neck. You then simply continue putting your hands in a straight line down the front of the torso, beginning with one hand over the thyroid at the hollow at the base of the throat and the other hand just below it over the thymus which is midway between the thyroid and the heart. Next, I place both hands over the heart, then both hands over the solar plexus, navel, and the belly and ovaries for women (above the pubic bone) and inguinal nodes for men when treating another. Men should treat the gonads directly during self treatment because it helps prevent prostate problems. After the "circular headband" positions on the head, and the straight line down the center, you can then treat the liver (to the right of the solar plexus), the spleen/pancreas (to the left of the solar plexus), and the upper lungs (these last positions form a perfect square). I teach the positions this way to make them easy to remember, but they also can be given in a different, more systematic order. Thus, the student need only remember: a circle around the head, a line down the front, and a square at the top and bottom corners of each rib cage.

Mrs. Takata placed a lot of importance on covering the heart, lungs, spleen, pancreas, liver, gallbladder, large and small intestines etc. on the torso after first completing the head. I complete treating the front of my body by letting Reiki be drawn into my knees and feet, and then begin on the back by treating my shoulders. With careful placement of the hands you can then treat your own kidneys, adrenals, lower back, and sacro-iliac crest. When treating another you can of course cover more of the upper back.

To treat specific ailments is quite simple. Mrs. Takata

always recommended a basic full body treatment if you have the time (and if you believe you don't, it's good to make time) in order to support the whole organism and put everything in balance. She would then do an extra 30 minutes on the problem area. For example, in the case of a tumor, she would treat directly over the tumor. In the case of arthritic joints, after a full body treatment, she would treat for an additional 30 minutes on the affected joints. With asthma, she would give extra treatment to the bronchial tract and so on.

It is essentially basic common sense: you give a minimum of an extra 30 minute treatment to the affected area. In addition, I suggest giving extra treatment to whatever position drew a lot of energy during the full body treatment, or to spots that felt particularly cold. Disease in one area of the body can sometimes be related to energy blocks in other areas, and through the vehicle of the full body treatment, you can easily discover them.

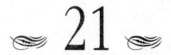

How do I know when to change positions?

Very simply, after three to four minutes, if there is no significant energy drawn, you will probably get an intuitive sense to move on. Because the body is warm throughout, it is natural that overall you will often feel a certain equal sensation of warmth.

Occasionally though, your hands may feel additional warmth, or even a hot tingling sensation or pulsation, or even an intuitive sense that the energy is being drawn. When this occurs, you want to leave your hands on that position for a longer period, until the sensation seems to dissipate. As long as you feel increased heat or sensations, this means an increased amount of energy is being drawn. This is why you want to keep your hands in this position until the sensation decreases. Also, one common occurrence is that when you are treating someone else, they will very often take a deep sigh (almost like a sigh of relief) when a certain position is complete. You can then move on.

If you find a cold spot, you may want to remain longer until the energy block "melts" and it begins to draw heat. Then wait until the drawing of the energy again seems to dissipate somewhat.

Overall I do not suggest timing the hand positions or necessarily treating particular positions for specific ailments. It is best to simply follow the body's own needs as revealed by the sensations in your hands, or a more subtle knowing (or instinct) which just tells you when one position is complete, thus a certain physical sensation is not absolutely necessary.

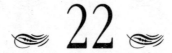

22

How long does it take to do a full body treatment?

In my First Degree classes I give my students 40 minutes on the front and 20 minutes on the back to complete one full body treatment. This is mainly due to my own time constraints.

I have found over the years, when I treat people without watching the clock, and simply follow the messages in my hands, my full body treatments seem to average anywhere from one hour and fifteen minutes, to an hour and a half. There is no harm in giving a longer or a shorter treatment. It all depends on the body's needs. Furthermore, if needed (such as in the case of cancer or AIDS) several treatments every day may be called for.

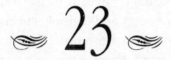

Is it OK to just treat the area which really needs it?

Yes, of course, everything depends on your own time constraints. Overall I encourage my students to simply trust their own intuitive abilities, to trust that first impulse in the moment which is usually correct. Although full body treatments with additional Reiki in the specific problem area are the ideal, when you have only a short time, Reiki given directly to the affected area is always beneficial.

~ 24 ~

Can I take on the other person's negativity or illness when I treat them with Reiki?

With Reiki it is virtually impossible to take on another person's negativity or illness, or for them to take on yours. In other forms of energy healing where you use your own reservoir of electromagnetic energy and transmit it to another, this might occur. Reiki, however, is Universal Life Force Energy which is channeled and drawn *through* you, *not* from you. From this you can logically conclude that the other person doesn't take on any of your personal energy patterns (physical or emotional stuckness), and likewise you don't take on theirs.

Occasionally you may treat someone who for example may be repressing a lot of grief and sadness. If you happen to hold similar emotions in your own body, in other words something in you is resonating on the same frequency as in the other person, you may start to process your own grief or sadness.

It is important to remember that as you give a treatment, you simultaneously also receive one. Consequently, you will sometimes feel joyful and refreshed after giving a treatment. At other times you may feel tired or somewhat down, especially if you haven't had enough rest, or if you begin to process some of your own previously repressed feelings. A consistent feeling of tiredness may also denote a low level chronic depression which may not even have been recognized as such. Depression is not a feeling in itself, but a repression of feeling. Such repression generally manifests as a feeling of fatigue or tiredness in the body. The body may then actually need to sleep off all the density of the stuck feelings, and Reiki treatments will act to induce the rest which is needed. The other way to deal with these feelings, is to simply feel them fully, consciously. (See *Abundance Through Reiki* and *Core Empowerment* for further clues on how to deal with stuck thoughts and emotions.) Ultimately, Reiki always gives you exactly what is needed to create balance both in yourself and others.

Another point to consider is, naturally, when you sit in the presence of another person, if you are open or sensitive, you may feel his or her feelings. Also, if you are very empathic (have the ability to truly feel with another) you may even perceive their physical pain.

These sensations are transitory however, and will quickly pass through the body if you approach your treatments on others with the attitude that you are there solely to support them in their process, (not to play the great "healer"). If you are not identified with the concept that you have to heal them or make them "better", such sensations will simply pass through. These sensations can be viewed as practical diagnostic tools which help you discern where to focus your attention during a treatment.

A simple way to deal with empathetic sensations of another is to thank the universe for the information, and then say "cancel, cancel, cancel". By acknowledging the sensations and not resisting them, they can be easily dissipated. When we say "cancel, cancel, cancel", we let go off any identification with the sensations, further acknowledging their transient nature, by not allowing them to become a "problem" to be fixed.

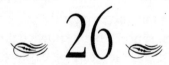

What do I have to do to make sure that Reiki flows?

The only thing you have to "do" to make Reiki flow, is have the *intention* to share it. Reiki basically happens on its own, as soon as you create the intention. Once it is flowing, there remains nothing to be done, except to simply listen to your hands, because they let you know through the sensation of heat, tingling, pulsation, or an intuitive knowing that the energy is still being drawn. For the few people who have very little kinesthetic sensitivity (are not feeling oriented, but may be more audio or visually oriented), I always recommend a lot of practice on many different bodies in order to develop kinesthetic sensitivity. Through the feedback from many others, you will eventually develop your own special sensitivity and know just when the energy is actually being drawn and when it has ceased to be drawn. Likewise, you will sense exactly when the time has come to change positions.

What should I think about when I give a treatment?

Once you have formed the intention to share a treatment and have begun the process, there is nothing to think about. Reiki is a listening process. Because Reiki just happens of its own accord, you ideally become like the captain of a ship who adjusts his course according to all the weather signals he receives. In the case of Reiki, the signals are either the sensations you feel in your hands and on your own or the other's body, and also sometimes just an intuitive sense that it is time to move on to the next position. There is a basic course you follow, but at times you will just know that you need to stay in one position longer than in another.

For beginners who find it difficult to simply listen, because the mind is still very active, focusing on the attitude of gratitude (one of the five Reiki principles) is very helpful. You can focus on gratitude for being able to act as a channel to either yourself or another of Universal Life Force Energy. You can then translate this attitude into your entire life as you go about your day. An attitude of gratitude fosters a very positive outlook on life. Many benefits accrue as a result, for as you focus on gratitude for what you have, you continue to stay in the state of having (rather than not having).

If you are distracted by too many random thoughts, don't resist them, simply allow them to pass through. Let them appear and disappear of their own accord. Don't argue with them. As you put all your attention on them *without trying to make them go away*, you'll be pleasantly surprised at the result.

27

Can I hurt someone with Reiki?

Absolutely and unequivocally: NO! As Reiki is *drawn* not sent, you do not really "give" Reiki; you only act as a vessel for the exact amount that the other person draws as needed through your channel.

It is very important to understand this, because occasionally you may give a person a treatment who seems to be in perfect health, but who after the treatment, actually feels worse than before. Very often people have problems brewing under the surface that they are not aware of, which Reiki brings to the fore to help heal.

In other words: Reiki can seem to exacerbate a problem before it gets better because it sometimes can create a short healing crisis, much like any of the natural healing arts which act to support the immune system and not suppress it. Once after doing a long lower abdominal Reiki treatment on an old friend who I knew had years before suffered from ovarian cysts, I received quite a surprise. Later that evening, she ended up in the emergency room of a local hospital in dire pain. As it turned out later, she had kidney stones she hadn't been aware of. The Reiki treatment, having accelerated her life force energy, had acted as an assist in passing the kidney stones and put her into a painful healing crisis. Such incidences occur occasionally, so it is important to remember that you cannot actually hurt any one in the sense of doing harm. Reiki only always helps to bring balance and healing, albeit sometimes through a healing crisis.

28

Can I give too much Reiki?

Because Reiki is always *drawn* not sent, you can never give too much Reiki. It is the idea of "giving" a Reiki treatment which creates this kind of misunderstanding. The body/mind of the recipient always knows instinctively what it needs and draws in just the right amount. No thinking is involved with either the Reiki channel or recipient during treatment, as Reiki far transcends the mind. Only the mind can worry about "giving too much Reiki".

The only thing that is necessary on the part of the person channeling the treatment, is attention or awareness focused on the hands, or on a sixth sense or intuition which just tells you when a position is complete. Even if you leave your hands on a position longer than the energy is drawn at a certain place, you can do no harm because the energy is again, only *drawn* in the amount as needed.

29

How long should I leave my hands on each position?

There is no set amount of time to leave your hands on any position. Essentially, if you have the time available, you should keep your hands in each position for as long as the energy is drawn. This could be three to five minutes, or in some positions even 30 minutes. It sometimes takes two to three minutes just to begin to feel the energy being drawn. In cases where chronic ailments are present such as a severely rheumatoid arthritic joint, it may take even 5 minutes or more before the energy really begins to be drawn and then you may experience intense heat or tingling for quite some time.

The key is to decide which positions on the body are most important to cover in terms of treatment, in the time you have allotted.

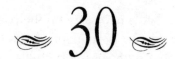

Why is it that someone occasionally may feel worse rather than better after a treatment, or even jittery or nervous during a treatment?

Sometimes when receiving a treatment, old feelings which have long been suppressed may come up and make a person feel antsy or nervous during the treatment. This happens more often when treating men, who are unfortunately conditioned to suppress their feelings. Hyperactive or aggressive A-type personalities often are overcome by a sense of uneasiness during their first treatment. The best thing to do then is to simply suggest that the person put all their attention on the jitteriness or uneasy feeling, allowing it to be there, without resistance. Continually direct them to just keep noticing the feeling (until it simply dissipates). However, do *not* tell them it will dissipate because this would set up the expectation that the sensation will disappear, which in and of itself is resistance to the jitteriness: it would then just become more entrenched.

In cases when actual physical pain is evoked, this is an indication that something has been there all along, but just had not yet surfaced until the time of treatment. Further treatments should then be given to help heal whatever has been brought to the surface. If the pain persists even then, a medical check up is in order.

≈ *31* ≈

Should I pray or do a mantra or some ritual before beginning a treatment?

It is helpful before beginning a treatment on either yourself or another to quiet your own mind. Although the act of sharing a treatment will eventually quiet the mind in and of itself, it is good to get into the habit of centering yourself so that you do not continue to dwell on the chattery thoughts which typically possess peoples' minds. Whenever you are lost in your thoughts (identified with them), you are basically fast asleep, because you are dwelling in memory so you are disconnected from the present moment.

The practice of Reiki on oneself or another, helps to bring you out of a state of unconsciousness and into the present. People who are used to prayers or mantras may find them helpful to center. Another useful way to center is to simply draw your attention to your heart. The centering meditation in *Empowerment Through Reiki* (p.95) is very helpful in drawing the focus away from the usual busy thinking mode right into Heart.

Another way to quiet the mind and connect with the person you are treating (even if it is yourself) is to begin noticing their breath and begin to breathe in synchronization with them. This helps to put you in the proper listening mode for Reiki and helps to pacify the mind.

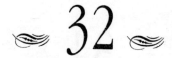

What should I focus on when treating myself or others?

The development of an attentive listening mode is the most essential ingredient for increasing your acumen as a Reiki practitioner. As was mentioned in answer to the previous question, centering at the very beginning of a treatment will help put you immediately in an attentive, wakeful stance. Bringing your attention to your heart for a couple of minutes and then shifting your attention to the other person's breathing, and eventually breathing with them, is a good way to begin.

There are several benefits to breathing in synchronization with the person you are treating. First of all it helps you to feel their feelings, it builds a sense of empathy as you begin to align with their energy pattern. In addition, because you are actively focused on their breathing, your own mind goes quiet and you can better sense their needs. Another benefit of synchronizing your breathing with the other person is that all the micro movements your hands make while touching them, fall into synchronization with their own subtle body movements. (All of a person's body movements are synchronized with the breath.) A sense of oneness occurs to the degree that the other almost always forgets your presence and falls into a deeper sense of relaxation very quickly.

Overall the most important focus to develop during Reiki is pure and simple awareness of what is. By using Reiki time as an opportunity to practice being present, the mind becomes increasingly quiet. A strong sense of peace and quiet then begins to carry over into the rest of your life as well. Stress decreases, and worry which is related to future and thus past concerns, begin to dissolve as you are more and more drawn into the present. Whenever you are focused in a true present, dis-ease is totally absent.

≈ *33* ≈

If Reiki is mainly for self treatment, why do you ask beginning students to do so many treatments on others for the first 21 days?

It is true, the best gift you can give to yourself or the planet is to work on yourself. When you are happy, it is easier for those around you to also be happy or free of stress. The reason why I suggest to my students the importance of treating many others in the beginning, is partly so that you gain clarity about the efficacy of Reiki. As you receive verification from all the people you treat, if some time later weeks or months go by and you find that you haven't made time to practice, you will have no trouble taking it up where you left off. You in effect will have no doubt about your ability to convey Reiki.

The other very important benefit of treating other people in the beginning, in addition to doing your own self treatments is that, due to our mind's subject/object relationship with the world, it is easier to focus on another person (an outside "object") and have your mind go quiet enough to notice what is happening in your hands. Typically, beginners complain of not noticing so much happening when they treat themselves as when they treat another. This is because we are so used to identifying with our chattery mind and its outward directed focus.

Most people find it difficult at first to lay their hands on themselves and just listen. They get distracted by the mind as it begins to think about all the things that didn't get done that day or what they need to do tomorrow. In truth, many people are fearful of just focusing on themselves and being quiet. They are often fearful of feeling long suppressed feelings and desires. By working a lot on others in the beginning, many of these worries get treated automatically, and it then becomes easier to just be with yourself and enjoy Reiki in peace and quiet.

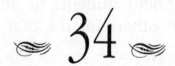

What is the 21-day cleanse process?

It takes about 21 days for the body/mind to assimilate the

attunements after each of the degrees. Because the attunements raise the life force energy on a cellular level in addition to opening the Reiki channel, often physical toxins are released as well as "toxic" emotions. In other words the body/mind is released of its density as it shifts into a higher vibratory frequency. None of the adjustments should be feared, as each person only experiences what he or she is ready for. Overall there is a sense of a lightening of energies on a physical as well as mental level.

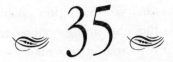

What are some of the reactions to the attunements ?

Most people feel a deep sense of relaxation during attunements, In a few, tears flow as many feelings are released from the heart. Occasionally some people may hear or see things such as sounds or colors, but there is nothing to be afraid of. I always advise my students also not to be disappointed if various phenomena do not occur, because this is definitely not important. Psychic phenomena or powers are never an end in themselves. If they were, they would only serve to inflate the ego beyond proportion. What is important, and is easily palpable after the attunements, is the amount of increased energy that is drawn through the hands.

36

Why do you ask us to keep a journal for the first 21 days after receiving the attunements ?

During the 21 day cleanse process a quickening occurs in the body/mind. As the life force energy is shifted to a higher, more loving frequency, what you have previously experienced as negative or dense thoughts and emotions are released. It is beneficial to keep a journal at this time to record whatever occurs.

It is important that you do not censor what comes up during your spontaneous diary session. Remember, the point of journal writing is *not* to describe beautiful events and happenings. You only have to write down what is passing through you at the moment, as truthfully as you possibly can, without embellishment, and with all the feelings and emotions this evokes in you.

Journal writing helps draw your attention to the old patterns which come up so that they can finally be let go of. Very often, the simple act of noticing one's own emotional or mental patterns rising up, and the ego then acting them out, diminishes their power over us with time.

≈ 37 ≈

Why do you recommend writing down our dreams during the 21-day cleanse process?

In addition to keeping a journal of the various things that happen to you during the day, and most especially your reactions to them, it is also helpful to record your dreams. Dreams are a wonderful reminder for helping us get in touch with what is hidden in the subconscious mind. The subconscious mind carries many of the aspects of ourselves that we tend to forget or unconsciously deny. In order to effectively "lighten our load", it is helpful to bring these hidden aspects into full awareness. On many spiritual paths, including the Native American and Tibetan traditions, conscious dreaming is considered a direct way to full realization.

Due to the acceleration of the vibratory frequency of the body/mind as a result of the attunements, many revealing dreams occur. To recall your dreams it is helpful to give yourself the suggestion every night just before you retire: "I will remember my dreams." Say this three times to yourself each night before falling asleep.

The first week you may only remember your dreams once or twice. By the second week you will remember them almost every day. It is important to write them down immediately upon awakening, so keep a pen and paper right by your bed. What is most important to note is your reaction to the events in the dreams. For example, when a man dreams about a woman, the woman most often represents some of the man's own feminine aspects. Similarly, when a woman dreams about a man, the role the character in the dream plays, speaks of issues she is dealing with in regard to the male aspects in herself. (You can also view the approach you take to the opposite sex in your daily life in the same way.)

Although some dreams can seem very abstract, it is important to still note them down. If you review your dreams after a month's time you will begin to perceive certain patterns in them. Intuitive insights will occur as you begin to get in touch with parts of yourself which have long called out for recognition. It is not only negative aspects which are revealed, what often arises are positive features which we are afraid to acknowledge due to false or negative conditioning.

You can also continue your dream journal after the 21-day cleanse process is over as well as your daily self treatments. This will support further self-observation and an increased awareness, leading quite naturally to a further refinement of your energy.

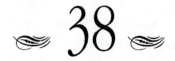

Is Reiki only for sick people?

Most definitely not. On the contrary, Reiki is one of the best preventative "medicines" on earth. It is recommended that you use it with the attitude of maintaining health rather than waiting for something to go wrong. Of course, if you or another friend or relative fall ill, Reiki can be used to amplify the life force energy and induce healing.

As Dr. Usui himself stated: Reiki heals indirectly by calming the mind and raising the life force energy. Because all of us suffer from some form of mental stress or physical discomfort, if used frequently, Reiki will eliminate the cause of stress which generally leads to physical illness.

THE FIVE PRINCIPLES

≈ 39 ≈

What are the five principles and where do they originate?

As an advanced Buddhist practitioner, Dr. Usui worked intimately with twenty-six moral precepts which he used in his daily healing practice as a physician. As these were a bit complex for simple lay practitioners, Dr. Usui adopted the Meiji emperor's five principles which he had given to the Japanese people to help improve the quality of their lives. Dr. Usui probably recognized the spiritual nature of the emperor's principles and how, if used wisely, they would remove the cause of suffering and disease.

In order to change a person's situation in life, there has to be a change in attitude, for whatever you think you will become. One bit of additional information I always share with my students is the fact that the universe is very generous: it will always prove your beliefs true. So, beware of what beliefs or concepts you adopt!

If followed faithfully, these principles will lead to a more positive outlook on life because, although at first mere concepts and beliefs, they are totally wholesome and life affirming when integrated. With a shift to a better attitude, greater abundance in the sense of a feeling of deep satisfaction and well-being is most often the result.

40

The first principle is: "Just for today I will be in the attitude of gratitude." What does it mean? How can the attitude of gratitude affect my life?

If we foster the attitude of gratitude until we become gratitude itself, life becomes a never ending expression of abundance. Whenever we concentrate on what we don't have (as many human beings do), we continue to experience the state of not having. Even if your life is currently to all appearances in a "negative" or down cycle, if you gather your resolve and begin to focus on all of the good things in your life: your family, the beauty of nature, your education, your talents etc. a shift will begin to occur.

The greatest challenge is to maintain the attitude of gratitude when things are not going well. My own remedy is to thank the God Force for allowing me to experience the body/mind's karma now, rather than in the future. Besides, a sense of humor will get you everywhere!

Also, don't forget to be in gratitude when things are going well because it is important not to become complacent and take things for granted. When you use gratitude with a sense of wonderment for the miracle of life that you are, you will stay forever young (even when the body/mind gets old or is cycling dis-ease!).

~ 41 ~

The second principle is: "Just for today I will not worry." How can I keep from worrying? How will freedom from worry affect my life?

Worry is a signpost which shows how stuck you are in the ego and its attachment to having things its way. It is one thing to have concern about our loved ones, or about taking care of business properly, and so forth. It is quite another to find that you are incessantly in worry mode. If this is the case for you, it is time to take stock, for you have essentially lost your faith and trust in the universe: you have forgotten who you are.

To worry is to forget that the body/mind is only an actor in a play which has always already been written. However, this doesn't mean we should just sit back and let life "do it to us". As a matter of fact, we *are* here to *participate* (with enthusiasm). Most of all, we are also here to enjoy and learn from the character we are called upon to play. Once we realize we are the dreamer or the playwright itself, all worry ceases.

Worrying over the past is futile. It is important to remember that each person (including yourself) does the best they can with the knowledge and life experience they have accrued in any given moment. Each person is a product of their conditioning. If you regret something you've done in the past feel your remorse fully until it dissipates, simply apologize and move on. Do not get into guilt or let anyone else lay that on you. Know that you act according to your resources, be thankful for every lesson and let go. Give everyone else the same credit.

Worrying about the future is also a total waste of time. I have a saying I shared ten years ago and still live by: Expect the best in life, and when you receive something you didn't expect, know (trust) that it is the best in your present situation. All of life's occurrences are only situations magnetized by the body/mind to learn from. Your body/mind has karma, but since you are not the body/mind (and thus do not have karma), what is there to worry about? Simply stay quiet and observe the one who worries.

꩜ 42 ꩜

The third principle is: "Just for today I will not anger." Does this mean that I should suppress my feelings? How do I avoid not getting angry?

Anger is another signpost that you are hooked by the ego. Anger arises when the ego notices things are not happening its way. Ironically, the best way to deal with anger is *not* to suppress it. Instead of getting angry at yourself for being angry, just stop and observe your anger (without trying to make it go away). Allow it to be there and just put all your attention on it. You can even imagine it as the ball of energy it is, and allow it to expand. Since your anger has a limited energy field, eventually it will dissipate. However, never try to use this technique with the intention of getting rid of the anger: it won't work. The moment you want to get rid of it, you will then be resisting the anger. And as we all know, whatever you resist, persists.

Anger is simply another bad habit of the non-existing ego. It comes up when there is fear. The best way to dispel it in another is not to react to it. (This does not mean ignore it because that is also a reaction.) When someone attacks you verbally, it might be better to ask them (with genuine concern): Are you OK? Did you have a bad day? Rather than going unconscious and reacting back automatically yourself, by taking the attack personally, you can instead observe the fear in the other which has caused the anger to arise. You can also do the same when your own anger comes up.

When anger arises it is important to feel it fully, and not judge yourself for it, or make it wrong. Repressing anger or rage only causes tumors or depression. By feeling it fully and putting all of your attention on it without trying to make it go away, we ultimately take the charge out of it.

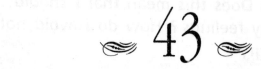

The fourth principle is: "In your daily work be honest (true) to yourself." How are we supposed to understand this?

This principle is essential, as it points out the importance of spending your time wisely in such a way that is true to your own heart. It addresses the need to choose a vocation which helps you grow, and provides you with a sense of fulfillment. It also infers that you need to speak your truth wherever possible and not be afraid to ask for what you need (even though there is always the chance you may get rejected). Eventually, you'll get it.

To be true to yourself also speaks to each individual's need to draw the bottom line, to not let others invade your emotional and mental space (sometimes even physical space) without your permission. Most important, it also addresses every person's need to take time for themselves. To be quiet and to enjoy your own company periodically, without interruption, is essential for maintaining a peaceful existence. Only *your* heart knows what is most appropriate for you. Thus, you need to honor its message, which only is audible in stillness, when you are quiet.

A walk in nature, time alone practicing an instrument or hobby, or even daily self treatments, can become that special time to just be by yourself. Ultimately, the more we are willing to give to ourselves, the easier it will be to give to others in a natural heartfelt way. Life is simpler, when we are true to ourselves.

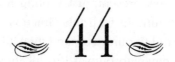

The fifth principle is: "Just for today, I will be kind and respectful to all of creation." What does this mean? What are the ramifications?

Due to quantum physics, science has finally grasped the fact that not only are living beings such as humans, animals, plants and trees, vibrant and dynamic, but so are rocks, minerals, air and water. In a direct sense, everything in creation is alive.

When students ask me in my class how you can give Reiki to a car or a toaster, I always point out that a car or different forms of machinery are simply extensions of our own body. The body itself is our vehicle for expression in this world (even though we ourselves are not the body), which is directed by the consciousness that we truly are. The tools we use regularly even take on our etheric energy and become extensions of the body. Did you ever notice how your car, computer, or toaster have the tendency to always break down when you are in a negative mental cycle, when everything seems to be going wrong?

This is because, in effect, we are all telekinetic like Uri Geller who bends spoons with his mind. After tuning in and bending a few spoons with my own mind years ago, I got the point. When we are out of synchronization mentally (because we are not listening to Heart) everything around us, including the physical body suffers. Love is the dynamic force that truly runs the universe. It is our choice to notice and act it out.

Grace is always present, just waiting for us to receive it. The best way to tune in with this Grace is to begin by being kind and respectful to ourselves, and then allow the effulgence of this Love to emanate outward to all those around us and to creation Itself.

45

How can I best use the five Reiki principles?

After I received the First Degree attunement, I used the first principle during every treatment I shared. I focused on the attitude of gratitude for being able to act as a channel to support another. So many positive shifts occurred in my life after First Degree, it was easy to focus on gratitude while doing self treatments. This became my time to focus on and appreciate all that is good in my life. I feel that as a result of this focus, an incredible amount of Grace began to flow, or a better way of putting it would be to say, I then began to notice (and thus manifest) what had been there all along. Even if challenging or unpleasant karmic episodes would arise, I now had the Grace to handle them with equanimity.

With the other four principles, I found it handy to put one each week on my bathroom mirror just to remind myself to notice when I either became angry, worried and so forth. I recommend changing the principle on the mirror each week, otherwise it begins to blend in with the scenery and you just go back to being unconscious.

The key to these principles, is that they can be used as powerful wake up tools: But you have to pay attention to them.

ALL ABOUT HEALING
WITH REIKI

$$\iff 46 \iff$$

Is Reiki more than a healing method?

Yes, as the title of the ancient Buddhist manuscript from which Reiki is derived illustrates, Reiki can be the first step toward realizing Self or Buddha Nature. *The Tantra Of The Lightening Flash That Heals The Body And Illumines The Mind* inspired Dr. Usui to create a simple system so that all lay people could treat themselves. The main focus of the tantra, as it is with all tantric work, is direct realization for the sake of all beings. In order to be able to work on oneself and realize the ultimate, good health and a strong mind are required.

It is difficult to attend to spiritual growth and development if your attention is focused on a sick or disabled body/mind. It is no wonder then that the synthesis of this ancient teaching, which Reiki is, deals with maintaining and/or regaining physical and mental health.

～ 47 ～

How does Reiki affect the body/mind ?

Dr. Usui expressed it best himself when he commented about Reiki, the synthesis of the ancient Tantric teaching for lay people: "What has been transmitted is only the pacification which is called the Soothing Hand, the healing. It helps to pacify, heal and soothe, but there is much more beyond this simple technique. It does not address the activity of healing in a direct manner. It addresses it in an indirect manner by increasing the body's energy, by relaxing the nervous tension of the body, and pacifying the upsets and imbalances."

～ 48 ～

How does Reiki affect chronic problems ?

Most pathologies fall into either of two categories: acute or chronic. Chronic problems, by definition, are physical or psychological symptoms which have gone on for quite some time. When you treat chronic problems, it may take a while before you feel the energy being drawn. Usually after a few minutes a strong heat or tingling may be felt in the hands, and in the case of painful arthritis for example, the person often describes a sensation of the pain rising to the surface and diminishing.

With chronic cases, people generally feel a whole lot better after one or a series of at least three treatments. Generally a healing crisis happens much later or not at all during an extended course of treatment. If a healing crisis does occur and the person describes an amplification of the problem, it is a good idea to do extra treatments at that time because this is a sign that the last vestiges of the disease are being released, and Reiki will speed up the process. In my first book, I referred to this type of occurrence as "physical chemicalization", because in effect, the body is burning up whatever toxins are left, in connection with the disease.

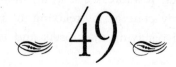

How does Reiki affect acute problems?

Acute problems are by definition of short duration: something has just risen to the surface and made itself painfully known. Ideally, an acute problem should be checked out by a qualified physician or naturopath immediately, however, if none is available and you are it, it is best to know what to expect.

Often when dealing with an acute problem with about any kind of natural medicine, including Reiki, treatment may initially exacerbate the pain (as usually the person is already in pain), rather than give immediate relief as in the case of chronic problems. Reiki sends so much powerful healing energy to the problem, Universal Life Force Energy will often be experienced as an irritation rather than a comfort.

It is important to realize this so that if a person complains, you can help soothe them by letting them know that this is actually a good sign that they feel a stronger sensation, as it shows that a lot of healing energy is being drawn. In acute problems, the pain will usually dissipate within two to three days. Again, it is important to remember that acute problems often produce more intense symptoms during the initial healing phase so that you can let the person know beforehand which enables them to adjust psychologically.

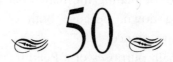

Do I have to remove my jewelry or clothes to either give or receive a treatment?

Absolutely not. Since Reiki is Universal Life Force Energy, as is everything else manifest in creation (including clothes and jewelry) how could Reiki block itself or interfere with itself? Some books have filled peoples' minds with a lot of nonsense about Reiki. In other forms of therapy such as Polarity it is important not to wear jewelry, but as Reiki is not magnetic (although it flows within magnetic parameters), there are absolutely no seemingly solid objects that it will not flow through. Reiki energy cannot be interfered with.

～ 51 ～

Is it OK to cross my legs, or for a person receiving a Reiki treatment from me to cross their legs?

There are no hard and fast rules about crossing limbs while treating with Reiki. Generally, I discourage people from crossing their legs or putting the hands back up behind the head while lying down, because both of these positions denote a protective stance.

One of the main purposes of a Reiki treatment is to calm the mind and help the person to feel their feelings. To feel your feelings, it helps to be in an open, "vulnerable" position. Crossing your legs while lying prone is a sign of discomfort or fear of vulnerability. It is actually helpful for the person to notice and feel their vulnerability. By putting all their attention on it, allowing it to be there, it will simply go through and disappear. My entire book *Core Empowerment* alludes to the true strength which lies in an open, vulnerable heart, which is contrary to what most of us have been taught.

When you remain true to Heart in open vulnerability you cannot be deceived, and neither can you be manipulated to unconsciously and blindly serve another's purpose. In other words, true to Heart, you will always fully live out the Truth that Heart is. You will not bend others to your will, but you will also not be subservient to theirs.

⚉ *52* ⚉

How long does it take to heal various diseases, and can I guarantee results?

There is no set amount of time for healing any disease, and absolutely no guarantee of results with any form of medicine, including allopathic treatments. All healing is pure Grace and just happens when the time is right. The best we can do when assisting another in their healing process, is to see them as totally perfect as they are (even if they have a disease), and trust that whatever process they are going through, is perfect for them, as it is all part of their learning process in life.

If we have a strong attachment to healing someone with our method (or any method) we actually do a disservice, as this sets up resistance in the other to receiving the healing. On the other hand, it is important to convey a clear and sure confidence to an ill person that they *can* indeed be healed. This is the greatest support we can ever give anyone, and is a sign of a true healer.

With the above all stated, there are average healing times for different diseases, but these are affected by the person's body/mind karma which is an unknown and by the person's willingness to change bad eating habits, and/or deal with long withheld emotions.

For example, in almost fifty years of clinical experience, Mrs. Takata noticed that small marble sized tumors would often disappear during two weeks of daily treatments (full body treatments, combined with an extra 30 minutes on the tumor). Mrs. Takata also recommended a change in diet, and a lot of freshly prepared carrot, beet and celery juice along with the treatments.

Basically she found, if a body part (for example as in spinal surgery) hadn't been surgically removed or messed with, sometimes even paraplegics could be cured. It really all depends on the person's openness to being cured. Ultimately, it is foolish to guarantee results. No doctor ever does. It is one thing to say with conviction: "You can be healed." It is quite another, to give guarantees.

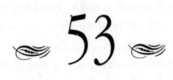

What is the optimal number of treatments to give another?

Mrs. Takata always insisted that whenever you started treating another person that you should try to give at least three treatments in a row. The first treatment seems to bring a lot to the surface on either a physical or emotional level. The second treatment acts to clear a lot out. The third leaves the body vibrant and filled with Universal Life Force Energy. It is good to do the three treatments over three consecutive days, or minimally within a weeks time.

Of course, if someone is suffering from a chronic ailment which has gone on for a long time, there will most likely need to be a longer series of treatments in order to see lasting results.

54

How long should I treat someone?

Basically, as long as they need it. After you have practiced Reiki for a while, you will begin to get an intuitive sense with people of how long they will need treatments, and you'll be able to make suggestions at the beginning as to how (approximately) many they'll need. Overall, chronic problems which have gone on for years may require weeks or months of treatments, whereas acute problems may only need a few.

Another factor determining how long a person will need treatments, is noticing if they are willing to give up the bad habits which contributed to creating the problem in the first place. For example, as in arthritis, are they willing to give up coffee, tea, dairy products and meat? If they have emphysema, will they quit smoking? And so forth.

When people refuse outright to make necessary changes which are related to the causal factor of their problem, I am very blunt in telling them that although Reiki may make them feel better for a while, they should not expect a complete cure from it or from any other form of medicine if they continue with their bad habits. One thing Reiki may help them with though, is in giving up the addictive habits or habit which lead to the disease in the first place.

Something else needs to be taken into account as well. Every once in a while you may work with a person for a long time who just doesn't quite get healed. It may be that the person is receiving some sort of secondary benefit from the disease (such as the attention they have long craved for), or that they are purely riding on your energy. If you sense someone is becoming co-dependent, and the healer-healee relationship is no longer healthy, it is wise to disengage and gently, yet with supportive input send them on their way. I usually tell such a person that I have assisted them in every way possible and that my intuition clearly tells me that the last step is up to them. I boost their self confidence with a great deal of encouragement, but clearly cut any apron strings of dependency.

≈ 55 ≈

Why should I charge for treatments or ask for an appropriate exchange of energy?

In Reiki, the cost is usually referred to as an exchange of energy. Considering that money and all other forms of exchange are basically different manifestations of energy, this is actually an accurate description.

Since Reiki is "a pearl of great price" it is important that it be appreciated (so that it is utilized). The first form of exchange of energy is to simply ask for something (to ask for help). This is necessary so that you are then open to receive what it is you need. Although it is hard for many people to accept this, the truth is, that almost everyone is attached to their suffering and in some way do not really want to let go of it.

The "non-existent" ego often prefers what it is familiar with, even if it happens to be a form of suffering. One example of this trend is people who choose one abusive spouse after another, or the person who dramatically tells you their troubles and tales of woe with a gleaming smile on their face. A person may in full "consciousness" claim to want to change, but their actions as they constantly go about sabotaging their happiness, often negate the claim.

I am not a cynical person, only a practical one, as I am sure Dr. Usui was. At a certain point, after spending years with helping people who only profess to need your help but lack the capacity and openness to really receive it, you begin to focus on the ones who really want it and are able to use it.

The people who seriously want help are number one, willing to ask for help (and really mean it), and secondly they are willing to offer something in return. This doesn't have to be money per se. In ancient times, and to some extent still today, it can mean totally letting go of money, such as in the case of a sadhu. This would be an appropriate exchange of energy for a multimillionaire for whom a normal sized fee would mean little or nothing. Giving up all attachment to wealth itself might be more of a challenge. With one of my students who did his Reiki master training with me, the exchange of energy was two exquisite and accurate copies of original Tiffany stained glass lamps which took him two years to complete. The amount of work he put in the lamps really helped him appreciate what he received. They are incredible works of art, and were truly a labor of love.

For most people, however, money is the most convenient exchange of energy, and there is no problem in setting an appropriate fee for what you have to share. The recipient will then more fully appreciate what you have to give them, and they are left free of a sense of obligation. The results they gain afterward is then dependent on their own effort.

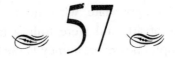

56

What kind of exchange of energy should I expect for sharing Reiki treatments?

When you treat people in your family or close friends, there is already a constant exchange of energy established, so there is no need, and it is probably not appropriate, to ask for one. If a neighbor you don't know very well hears about Reiki and asks you to help them, you can always offer a sample treatment. However, it is wise to let them know it is best to have three successive treatments, and then perhaps ask for an exchange of energy in the form of a suggested donation to yourself or your favorite charity, some favorite food you like (that they can prepare) or some such thing. This leaves them free of feeling beholden to you, and will help them further appreciate your time and effort. They also gain more benefit.

If you decide to offer Reiki to the public, you can set an appropriate fee, or ask for donations according to each person's ability to pay.

57

What should I do if I don't feel differences in different hand positions on the body?

If it is only on yourself that you don't feel differences, this is related to the fact that it is difficult for most people to stay quiet and really focus on themselves. Most beginners tend to get lost in their own thoughts as the chattery mind distracts their attention from what is happening in the hands. For these people it is still appropriate to do a lot of treatments on others, until the quiet mind you develop when focused outward on another finally begins to have an effect when you work on yourself.

If you also don't feel any differences when you are treating other people, this is probably due to the fact that you are not kinesthetically oriented. In other words, you may be more audio or visual in your orientation and not so body sensitive, such as in your hands. If this is the case, I recommend also doing a lot of treatments on others. Although you may not notice differences at first, some of the people you treat will give you feedback, which will eventually clue you in to the variations in your hands.

Eventually with practice, the synapses in your brain will begin to connect with the nerve endings in your hands, and you will begin to notice what may be for you, subtle differences in different positions. Also, with practice, your intuitive sense will develop and you will just know when to move to the next position, regardless of any physical sensations.

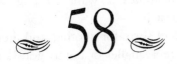

How can I develop empathy so that I can sense more what another needs?

In answer to question 31, I described a way of breathing in synchronization with another which will help you begin to feel what another is feeling. Our whole life revolves around the breath. When we are in our heart we tend to breathe with full deep breaths in the lower belly.

On the other hand, when we breathe shallow breaths in the upper chest, this can be taken as a clear sign that we are stuck in our heads and focused on our thoughts. Taking a few deep, full belly breaths and consciously filling out the lower abdomen and lifting the rib cage just before beginning a treatment, will help you to center and relax the mind.

We tend to tune into others better when we are focused in the heart, and in listening mode, rather than thinking mode. True empathy (feeling with another) happens more easily when we are quiet and open to receiving, rather than in a state of trying to figure out what another needs with the mind.

It is important to note the difference between empathy and sympathy, because too many so-called healers approach their "healees" with sympathy. Sympathy or feeling sorry for someone, because they have some awful problem or disease does not honor them. In any case, it would be actually more accurate to say *thinking* sorry, for sympathy does not involve real and unfiltered feeling. Sympathy is insidious, because it is a one upmanship game. In effect you, as (ego), put yourself above the other and feel pity for the "poor unfortunate creature" who is undergoing whatever they happen to be undergoing. Sometimes I want to gag when I see this missionary approach.

When you feel sorry for another and then buy into it, the other begins to feel smaller or not as good or capable as you. You actually help perpetuate their misery by supporting them in the victim role. You get to play "heap big rescuer dude" and pump up your ego — while they continue forever to play the miserable victim. It is a sickening self perpetuating merry-go-round.

Empathy, however, is something quite different. It takes a genuine open heart to feel empathy, because empathy involves the ability to truly feel with another (not think sorry thoughts about them). Practice putting your attention on the heart when you are treating and breathing with another, and you may begin to experience some amazing things.

When you approach each being with total equanimity, honoring their need to undergo whatever experience they are undergoing, the world takes on quite a different color. The secret is to turn this same approach around on yourself.

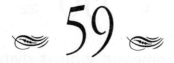

How can I protect myself against taking on another's pain?

The more awake you are, the more you also become sensitive to others' pain. At times, you may even feel their pain or emotion in your own body. The secret here is not to become identified with it. If you don't identify with it, it will simply go through. It is when you begin to buy into (believe in or identify with) the "big healer" role of believing you have to save the world (or even one person) and make him or her or the whole world *better,* that your problems start.

In actual fact the world is perfect as it is, even with all its many and blatant imperfections. We happen to be living at the end of the age of kal yuga (the densest of the four world ages), so sometimes it can get downright uncomfortable! The secret is not to be attached to feeling happy or sad, good or bad, but to notice the perfect silence behind all the noise of your mind (and of others' minds) and stay with that silence. You may then feel occasional unpleasant sensations pass through you as you move through your life, but they won't overwhelm you.

As you begin to develop greater sensitivity and first feel others' pain, you can thank the universe for the information (as it tells you where to place your hands or keep them longer) and then say "cancel, cancel, cancel", so you remember not to get hooked on it.

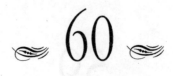

Can I treat someone who is dying?

Absolutely. Sometimes the greatest healing occurs during the death process. For anyone familiar with the *Tibetan Book Of The Dead*, the bardos or intermediary states at the time of death and for forty-nine days after death has occurred, provide a rare opportunity for self realization. Giving a dying person Reiki will help to calm their mind and give them an easier passage in a process which is not much different from birth. In fact, Reiki is also good for mother and child during the birthing process.

Once Mrs. Takata felt compelled to give Reiki to a friend's corpse at the heart area about half an hour after she had died. The woman came miraculously back to life just as they were bringing in the coffin to take her away! As I recall, the woman lived about five more years. Many amazing things have happened with Reiki. Whether it heals you of an ailment, or helps you through a difficult passage, it is of great benefit.

61

Can Reiki be used with other healing methods?

Reiki stands on its own as a self contained healing method. It does not need to be combined with any other technique to improve it. However, if you are already a practitioner of another healing art, you may choose to use Reiki with it. Many allopaths, homoeopaths, naturopaths, chiropractors, ayurvedic physicians, acupuncturists and massage therapists have found Reiki to be very beneficial with their patients. Its soothing and calming effect helps quell a patient's worries, fears and stress. The fact that Reiki raises the life force energy, it helps to indirectly improve the efficacy of any other healing method.

62

Will Reiki go through casts, metal and other hard objects?

Reiki will go through *anything*. Since Reiki is what everything is made of, and everything is Universal Life Force Energy, there is nothing that it cannot penetrate. As substratum itself, it can be drawn through casts, metal, and all seemingly solid objects, because as we already know, there is truly no solid matter.

⪻ 63 ⪼

Can I give Reiki to my car, computer, toaster or other inanimate object?

Because the different types of machinery we use are all extensions of the physical body, it is possible to give Reiki to them. Any clothes or objects you use constantly, begin to take on your etheric energy or imprint. It has been proven scientifically that 99% of disease is psychosomatic or caused by the mind. In truth any disease (including accidents) is 100% psychosomatic.

In the same way that our mind affects the body, our mind also affects the machines we use all the time. Just notice how often your car or computer screws up when everything in your life (mind) has gone awry. As in healing the body there are no guarantees, it is the same with these inanimate objects. However, I have had great success periodically with cars and a few assorted gadgets.

Much like taking care of the body by using Reiki as preventative medicine, you can Reiki your car or boat or computer to keep it in good shape. This is actually more preferable than troubleshooting under pressure when you need to fix something that has broken down.

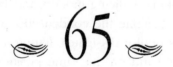

Can I do distance Reiki at First Degree level ?

While Second Degree Reiki focuses specifically on distance healing and amplifies the life force energy to do so, there is no reason you cannot try it at First Degree level. In my doctoral dissertation years ago I quoted a study done by a cardiologist on 100 of his patients who received bypass surgery. Fifty percent of the group (unbeknownst to them) were prayed for and fifty percent were not. The group who were prayed for did remarkably better. Recently, Larry Dossey wrote a whole book on the healing effects of prayer, called *Healing Words*. You can simply imagine a tiny image of the person in your hands and give them Reiki because, in a way, the sharing of Universal Life Force Energy is a silent and very beautiful form of praying for someone.

How can I use Reiki to remove energy blocks from the body ?

Occasionally when you are giving yourself or another person a Reiki treatment, you may come across a spot where the energy doesn't seem to draw, and it may even feel cool to the touch. This is generally a sign of an energy block, where a thought form and its corresponding emotion are stuck in the body. It is important to be aware that sometimes a point on the body may feel cool in relation to the heat in your hands, because in actual fact the person is drawing a lot of energy. So, you have to discern whether it is clearly an energy block or in actual fact your hands feel hot in comparison to the patients body temperature because he is indeed drawing energy. Sometimes asking yourself quietly will evoke a simple answer: yes or no, if you aren't sure.

Once you have determined that there is an energy block, by simply leaving your hands on long enough, the dense energy will begin to dissipate. If you have received Second Degree, utilizing the second symbol will help release the block. For First Degree practitioners there is a simple technique I teach, a sort of short cut which is not a Reiki technique, but which is derived from psychic surgery:

What you can do is scoop both of the hands together over the energy block and gather it into a tight compressed ball on the surface of the body. You can grasp it with your left hand and raise it away from the body. Then sever it with your right hand by making a slicing motion, totally disconnecting it from the body. Imagine the condensed energy expanding for a few seconds until it dissipates, letting it go totally, and then replace your hand on the same position. You will be surprised at how quickly the energy will begin to draw.

≈ 66 ≈

Why are so many people attracted to Reiki today?

There is a great need in every sentient being today to raise the vibratory frequency of life force energy. It appears to me that we are living at a time when tremendous love energy is engulfing the planet as we shift into a new and higher vibratory frequency. Unfortunately, when this higher vibratory frequency comes up against all the density stored in most peoples' bodies, it can cause a lot of pain or discomfort.

Most people are carrying lifetimes of grief and anger which need to come out and be released. Most feel drawn to this new energy and want to feel better at this higher frequency, but the higher frequency just acts to highlight their overwhelming sense of stuckness. This is one of the reasons we see so much strife in the world. Instead of safely pounding out rage on pillows, people are picking up guns to shoot it out on each other and adding fuel to the current ego explosion.

Fortunately, due to incredible Grace, Reiki has reappeared: a simple easy tool to raise every individual's life force energy so that this new frequency can be received joyously. Reiki not only raises the vibratory frequency, it also calms the overly distracted and scattered mind, the very root of all fear: the ego. The non-existent ego is turning rampant in its fear of extinction, in its "solid" sense of doership. With the Grace of Reiki and other such gifts, may it all implode with the ease of the Berlin wall!

In short, people everywhere on the planet are turning to

energy work such as Reiki because they are fed up with the deception and lies which are fed to them day in and day out. There is a great need for genuine empowerment, and Reiki puts you in touch with its source: the Heart.

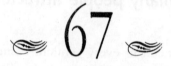

What is the best time to do Reiki ?

Anytime is Reiki time. There is no special time of the day to give "better" Reiki. It can be given before or after a meal, but it might be wise to let food settle a bit so that you have an opportunity to feel your feelings better. To make it easy on yourself you can do self treatments every night just when you lay down to go to sleep. I usually get as far as my brow and occipital lobes, or perhaps the heart, and then I fall asleep. In the morning I simply start where I left off. I then sit up and do my knees, feet and all the back positions.

It is helpful to do Reiki first thing in the morning and the last thing at night. You start your day with a quiet mind, and you finish in the same way.

≈ 68 ≈

What will happen to me after practicing Reiki for a while?

Most people experience a new feeling of vibrancy in their lives. The mind becomes less preoccupied, and a greater sense of peace is the result. I have had many grateful spouses tell me stories about a cranky husband or wife who after a few treatments with Reiki begins to behave like a much more loving human being.

People who have been ill or suffered chronic problems for a long time often experience great relief, and many are completely healed of their ailments. Cigarette smokers often find out that their desire to smoke just disappears. Overeaters and drinkers also undergo a waning of their addictive behavior, as simultaneously they are exposed to feeling their suppressed feelings which caused the addictions in the first place. These feelings then begin to be gradually released.

In the beginning there may be physical or emotional cleanse processes as the most dense energies are immediately sloughed off. However, these soon dissipate, as physical and subtle energies become more balanced.

~ 69 ~

What do I do if my life takes a bad turn after things have been going well for a long time?

This is a question I sometimes get from students who have used Reiki for three or more years. Things tend to improve immensely after the First Degree level as so many old negative patterns fade away. If Second Degree is used to its greatest benefit, by doing distant treatments on old childhood traumas and conditioning, the process of freeing up old behavioral tendencies continues.

At a certain point for most people a fear will arise which is something like: What will happen if all my patterns disappear? What will be left? This is an ego based fear which arises the more deeply the mind goes quiet.

The ego is in effect the biggest "possession" of all, even more so than a ghostly possession. It is what keeps the body/mind coming back again and again in different forms on the wheel of life as it reincarnates itself over and over.

As you get close to real freedom, the mind goes wild as it feels itself dissolving. It much resembles a dying fish in the throes of death, flopping all about. The more you get in touch with the unlimitedness of being, of that which you truly are, the ego can go manic (just observe the world today). As such, the ego doesn't even exist, as it is only a construct of the mind to help the body/mind survive in the world. Its fear of dissolution often gets projected on the outer world, and before you know it, things seem to fall apart for a while, as more of your fears manifest before you.

Since, by having seen through many of your patterns, you now have a more solid foundation however, the fear eventually begins to recede. One way it can be dealt with is to keep a vigilant observance on the "one" who fears. Continuous self inquiry will put the true culprit out of commission. For further handy hints on how to deal with this, the 42-day abundance plan in *Abundance Through Reiki* points out ways as to how to be vigilant in your daily life, and *Core Empowerment: A Course In The Power Of The Heart* gives you clues on how to live as Heart. Both of these books are recommended for those who want to live as Peace and Freedom.

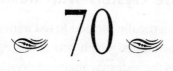

Should I use crystals with Reiki?

There are no shoulds and no shouldn'ts with the practice of Reiki. If you are drawn to both Reiki and crystals, you can refer to my first book, *Empowerment Through Reiki* which describes a variety of ways to use crystals.

Crystals have been used for centuries in different healing and spiritual traditions. It has now come to light with the discovery of Dr. Usui's own diaries, that crystals and various precious stones were used in the practice of Reiki. In the parallel Buddhist Tantric teaching of *Men Chhos Rei Kei* (which in English translation would read as "Medicine Teachings of Universal Life Force Energy") based on Dr. Usui's own practice, the use of crystals and charged elixirs are introduced at the Second Level. The crystals which act to amplify or maintain an energy vibration, are very often placed on the diseased area of a patient to help the body continue to draw energy.

Crystals act very much like batteries because they can store energy and information and then send it out in an amplified form, which is why they are so much part of modern information and other technologies.

❧ 71 ❧

How can I use crystals with Reiki ?

A crystal is a geometrically formed fused mineral or substance, with molecules or atoms which are arranged in a repeating pattern. This gives the external shape of crystals a symmetrical appearance. They have a stable geometrical and mathematical orderliness which they maintain with extreme precision, a factor that contributes to their usefulness as a programming tool. In *Empowerment Through Reiki*, I mentioned how their capacity to form and hold a specific energy matrix and transduce information between the subtle levels or planes of existence is another key to their usefulness as a healing tool. In other words, their usefulness lies in their ability to work primarily on the subtle energy bodies.

Most dis-ease in the body manifests first in the etheric or energy body. We can perceive these blocks with Reiki when we come across a cool spot or an area which doesn't seem to draw energy. After treatment, you can charge a crystal and leave it with the person to be used over the area that seems blocked. It will help to dissipate the blocked energy and charge the area with further energy.

The simple basics for using crystals are: to clear or cleanse the crystal; to charge the crystal; and if you want to expand its capacity, you can activate it. In addition, by focusing your positive thoughts, you can also program the crystal. The essentials are cleansing and charging the crystal which I will briefly explain here.

To clear or cleanse a crystal you can soak it in a salt water solution for 24 hours. Another method is to use running water, or also by blowing on each of their facets while visualizing them as clean and pure. To charge a crystal with Reiki, simply hold it between your hands with the intention of charging it, and then focus on the purpose for which you wish to use it. Then you simply give it to the person who needs it to carry in their pocket, or to place on the special area which requires extra attention.

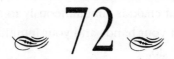

Is chakra balancing a part of Reiki, and if so, how do I do it?

Yes, indirectly. Mrs. Takata who brought Reiki to America, never focused on chakras per se. What she stressed over and over again is the need to treat the entire endocrine system as well as the major organs. It just so happens that the placement of the endocrine glands corresponds directly to the seven main chakras or energy centers.

The endocrine glands such as the pineal, pituitary, thyroid, thymus, adrenal and gonads keep the entire physical body in balance. Likewise, the crown chakra, third eye, throat, heart, solar plexus, belly and root chakras keep the etheric or energy body in balance. Both the endocrine glands and the chakras act as transducers, transmitting energy back and forth to the physical and etheric bodies.

One of the great benefits of Reiki is that it works both on the physical and the etheric bodies simultaneously. Also as you do a Reiki treatment and are open and sensitive enough to feel, you will pick up immediately if one gland or chakra is out of balance, because it will either draw an excess of energy in comparison to the rest of the body, or it may feel cool due to an energy block. Thus a full body Reiki treatment is really the best way to balance the chakras, as you'll feel just which area may need more energy.

If you wish to concentrate just on the chakras you can even have the person stand sideways in front of you, and then put one hand in front and one hand in back on each of the main chakras, and slowly move from top to bottom over each of them. You can also have the person laying down. Occasionally you may also get an intuition to put each of your hands on different chakras simultaneously to somehow create balance. Just trust your hands and your intuition, and they will tell you what to do.

Can Reiki protect me from negative energy?

The more you use Reiki, the more you also raise your life force energy automatically. As you raise the vibratory frequency of both your physical and etheric bodies, dense or "negative" vibrations can no longer enter. One good example of this very phenomenon is the experience many of my Second Degree students share when they describe what has happened to them after First Degree.

After doing a lot of self treatments and treatments on others, they notice that many old "friends" drift away and new ones appear in their life. The new friends are happier, more positive people. Only the old friends who are also happy, positive people themselves, tend to stick around.

One of the greatest benefits of Reiki is that it slowly teaches you that there is ultimately nothing you ever have to protect yourself from. As you mature spiritually you begin to understand that in truth there is no "good" or "bad", "right" or "wrong". There are only conscious people and unconscious people.

"Evil" deeds are done by people who are fast asleep, even though they may seem right on the ball and very cunning on the surface. If you are awake, with an open and vulnerable (feeling) heart, you will be able to sense the deep pain and anguish which drives people to hurt others. Although it definitely hurts to be on the receiving end, you will not take it personally if you are truly aware of the other person's motives.

Another essential point you need to be aware of, is that by buying into or accepting the concept that there are others that you have to protect yourself from, you immediately assume that others are more powerful than you. This then enables others to lay power trips on you, as they sense your fear unconsciously and act on it.

Of course, there are brutes in the world whom it is necessary to be aware of, thus you need to be vigilant all of the time: most of all to your own ego (which is what puts you in fear in the first place). Not even a magician of evil intent can harm a hair on your head, if you don't believe in his or her power.

With unconscious brutes who want to use sheer physical force, we need to learn to do some form of Aikido with them (i.e. learn to deflect their energy right by, or let it turn right back on themselves, or simply get out of their path). Sometimes, when such people become too overwhelming, they have to be dealt with. Very often it is best to baffoon them, to relegate them to their proper place. At that time, the superior intelligence of the heart will guide you. It will also tell you when the best thing you can do is confront them skillfully without hurting yourself (i.e.: by confronting them consciously without *internal* resistance).

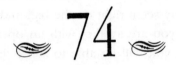

How can I center myself with Reiki?

By its very nature, Reiki has a centering effect. In *Empowerment Through Reiki*, I shared a lengthy centering process which focuses the attention and directs it away from the head into the *hara* (or *ki* or *chi* center) in the belly. Since in this almost totally westernized world educated people tend to identify with the intellect and its limited capacities, it is important to learn how to reconnect with your feelings which give a truer sense of the situation at hand. In martial arts, the belly or naval chakra has always been the focus for centering.

Although it is helpful to center in the belly, or *hara*, these days I find my attention focused on the heart. To me, it is most important to stay centered at all times in Heart, with THAT which we all are. Heart in this sense, goes way beyond the simple physical heart, or even the heart chakra. The Heart of who we truly are totally transcends all limits of time and space. At the Heart of who we are, time and space as we conceive or know them do not even exist.

As a human being with a body it helps to connect first with the physical heart, to lay your hands on the heart chakra and give yourself Reiki. As the heart stirs and the mind goes silent, you will begin to sense the longing, your very own heartfelt desire for that which you truly are. From this still small point there is no better guide or guru to the awesome nature of your real beauty.

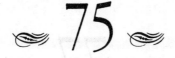

Can I do Reiki if I am already doing other spiritual practices or forms of meditation?

Yes, Reiki does not interfere with any other spiritual practice. It can only enhance it by raising your life force energy and relaxing any stress or nervous tension.

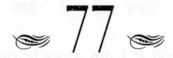

Can I mix Reiki with other forms of spiritual practice ?

It all depends on the practice. Some paths seem to be rather territorial and protective of their flock.

From the point of view of Reiki there are no objections whatsoever. If the practice calls for a calm or quiet mind, and you need more energy to do your practice, Reiki will be beneficial.

Reiki actually can be used as a spiritual practice in and of itself. Daily practice of Reiki helps you become a more loving, heart centered person which, in essence, is the core of any spiritual practice.

How does Reiki affect meditation ?

Reiki helps meditation by quieting the mind which usually talks a mile a minute. Reiki in and of itself could almost be called a form of meditation because, with practice, it silences the overly busy mind very effectively. Also, since Reiki is Heart energy, it helps you become a more compassionate human being: both towards yourself and others.

To my students who are meditators, I often suggest that while doing self treatment, they focus or meditate on the one who wants to meditate. This particular type of inquiry, if done with strong intent, can end all meditation because the meditator simply dissolves in direct self realization.

～ 78 ～

Can I mix Reiki with other forms of therapy?

Reiki stands on its own as a complete form of treatment, however it can be easily blended with different forms of body work or massage, rebirthing, and acupuncture or acupressure. It also works well with more mainstream forms of medicine. Psychologists may find it helpful as well, as Reiki can help people tune in with their immediate feelings. Also, although I don't generally recommend talking during a Reiki treatment, if emotions come up that a person needs to discuss, you can talk and still give Reiki.

～ 79 ～

Will Reiki have an effect on the use of allopathic drugs?

Yes, people generally need lower dosages the more Reiki treatments they receive. For example, very often doctors of diabetics who use Reiki, find that their patients need less and less insulin. Also, doing Reiki helps remove the craving for sugar itself which most often leads to diabetes in the first place.

⟫ 80 ⟫

Can I continue drug treatments while receiving Reiki?

Yes, the only thing is, you may need to monitor the dosage because you perhaps will need less due to Reiki's indirect beneficial effect.

⟫ 81 ⟫

Do I need to change my diet when I do Reiki?

I only ask students for the duration of my First or Second Degree class to abstain from coffee, tea, alcohol and heavy food. I also recommend that they minimize sugar intake, because all of these substances tax the body. Coffee, tea and sugar are addictive substances which have a deleterious effect on the nervous system. Since the attunements or empowerments of Reiki shift the vibratory frequency of the body, toxins are often released very quickly. You are asking for a more intense

21-day cleanse process if you keep putting toxins in your body. For people who are heavy tea or coffee addicts, I suggest "homeopathic" (smaller and smaller) dosages for a while. Going cold turkey (quitting too suddenly) could otherwise cause headaches and other cleansing reactions in addition to the possible cleansing effects of the attunements.

As far as diet is concerned, that is your own choice. When people are sick with cancer I generally recommend Gerson therapy which essentially is raw food diet. The raw live enzymes in raw vegetables and fruit act to boost the immune system. For example, even dogs when they are sick eat grass. Gerson therapy has been a proven cure for cancer for over seventy years. I actually cured myself of two tumors using it. The important thing is to make sure you eat or drink the freshly pressed juice of organically grown vegetables and fruit so that you don't put your system under additional stress from cancer causing residues of pesticides.

The longest lived peoples in the world are the Hunzas, Bulgarians, some tribes from the Caucasus and the Mayans. What they all have in common is that they all eat at least 75% raw foods, and often live to be 120 years old, some as old as 140! Most people today eat 95% cooked food, and even if it is good vegetarian fare, it is still dead food.

If you want to maintain your youthful vigor, healthy raw salads, bean sprouts and fruit are a good choice. Also, fasting twice a year for at least seven days on a combination of fresh lemon juice and equal parts of maple syrup or molasses or cane juice (no honey and absolutely no white sugar!!) mixed with water, you will feel truly rejuvenated. Refer to any of Paavo Airola's books for information on fasting.

ᕙ 82 ᕘ

Can I get rid of addictive habits like smoking or drinking with Reiki?

If there is a strong desire to quit there is an equally good chance for success. Paradoxically, I generally suggest to my Reiki students who really want to quit smoking, not to bother trying to quit. The desire to quit anything is resistance (to the addiction). You often end up smoking more because (as we all know) whatever you resist, persists.

Instead, what I generally suggest is to make a commitment to yourself to wait only five minutes every time you get an urge to smoke (or drink) and then allow yourself to smoke later if the urge is still there. Most often, what happens is that in the five minutes you wait, the feelings you were avoiding by smoking come up, so that the urge to smoke disappears. Treating yourself with Reiki also helps you to feel your feelings in a totally non-threatening way.

Basically all addictions are a simple avoidance of feelings (see in *Core Empowerment* for a more in-depth presentation of the connection between repression of feeling and addictions). When we learn to accept our feelings often the addictions simply vanish. This has happened to many Reiki practitioners who found that smoking simply became distasteful.

83

Will Reiki cure overeating and help me lose weight?

Overeating like all addictions is related to not wanting to feel certain feelings. There are two main motivations for most human actions: to feel something or to avoid feeling. If you are very much overweight and do not have a serious thyroid problem, chances are Reiki will assist you by at least helping you to feel your feelings.

The next step is to look at your diet. If you use any oil or butter (or ghee) you need to relearn how to cook. Try steaming food, rather than frying or boiling it, and experiment with non-fat, non-oily sauces. Barbecued or Tandoori style food is also less oily. If you cannot find a proper steamer, you can improvise with a steel colander in a larger pot. Add water to the pot until it reaches the steamer or colander, add your veggies and close the lid, and bring to a boil until they are still slightly raw.

The other handy hint for losing weight is exercise. When I'm on the road (which is a lot) I minimally do calisthenics: 200 sit-ups (start with fifty and work your way up); 100 leg-lifts to the side, inner thigh and lifting up from the back. At home, I do aerobics three times a week. I won't tell you how old I am, but I look and feel ten years younger than most people my age. A little discipline does pay off.

Once you get into the habit of exercise, you'll never want to stop because after fifteen minutes of exercising, the endorphins (the natural feel good "high" of the body) kick in, and all stress and worry simply disintegrate. Reiki, good diet and exercise are open secrets to a healthy body.

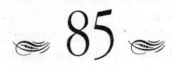

Are group treatments helpful?

Group treatments are a wonderful way to get together and share Reiki. Because several people work on each person, a full body treatment takes less time. Having a number of hands on the body also gives a great sense of comfort and support. I usually recommend to my students to arrange Reiki gatherings, because it's always enjoyable to be treated by someone else, or occasionally even by several other people simultaneously.

For these Reiki gatherings I also recommend finishing all the conversations first, and then turning on pleasant meditative style music to create a nice quiet calm atmosphere so that everyone is at peace and relaxed enough to feel the soothing presence of Universal Life Force Energy.

Can I treat plants and animals with Reiki?

Plants love Reiki, and I can attest to great success in my gardens both in Washington state in America and in the tropics in India. You can simply hold your hands up with palms facing the plant and let it draw.

Animals also enjoy Reiki. I have treated many dogs, cats,

horses and even snakes (not the poisonous variety). Basically you follow the same pattern of treatment on animals that you do on human beings.

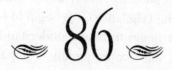

Can I treat my food with Reiki ?

It is very good to treat your food with Reiki. Simply hold your hands over your plate and let it draw. In the moment you Reiki your food, your mind also quiets down and it is easier to receive your meal to its greatest benefit. Treating food enhances it with life force energy, which unfortunately most food is lacking in these days, due to degeneration of quality from the approach of big agro business. Finally, when you have finished eating, you may also Reiki your belly to enhance the digestive process.

How does Reiki release old blocks and emotional or mental patterns ?

Reiki helps you feel the feelings which lie behind all surface emotions and general behavioral tendencies. As we are enabled to feel our deeper feelings, old habits and proclivities simply lose their hold. They may still sneak up on us for a while (old habits die hard) whenever we are tired or cranky from not eating or overworking, but are soon dissipated through the willingness to simply admit them. With practice and simple noticing (vigilance), we begin to take our patterns less seriously. We begin to finally understand how automatic they really are, and consequently compassion for both ourselves and others is the result.

SECOND DEGREE BASICS

~ 88 ~

What is Second Degree?

Second Degree Reiki is the next step in attunement to the Reiki energy. In addition to a further empowerment which helps to fine tune both the physical and etheric (energy) bodies to a clearer frequency of Universal Life Force Energy, certain symbols are also taught which enable the student to let Reiki be drawn across time and/or space.

Through the use of the Second Degree symbols, distant treatments can be shared with others. Additional tools are also given, to enable you to use distant treatments on yourself to release traumas from the past. These old energy blocks, if not attended to, could still continue to affect you in the present. At Second Degree level, your awareness is amplified to help you focus your attention so that you are enabled to address the root cause of disease: mental and emotional upsets.

❧ 89 ❧

How much or how long should I practice Reiki before taking Second Degree?

It is wise to use Reiki for a minimum period of three months. I even encourage my students to wait as long as six months and practice it consistently every day. After First Degree, it takes the body 21 days just to assimilate the four attunements. In certain (rare) circumstances Second Degree can be given after 21 days as I mentioned in *Empowerment Through Reiki*, but it usually is not in the students best interest.

The First Degree attunements accelerate the life force energy. Using Reiki continuously every day on oneself and others helps to keep the process going. The longer you practice Reiki the more you increase your vibratory frequency. Thus, the student who uses First Degree for a period of time will not only become fully familiar with its subtle nuances and be better prepared to use it, he or she will then also receive a proportionally greater boost with the Second Degree attunement.

Thus three to six months minimum experience at First Degree level is recommended. It should also be noted that some people who have actually waited a few years to receive Second Degree have noted major openings as a result of their thoroughness and patience.

90

How many attunements are there in Second Degree ?

In Second Degree only one attunement or empowerment is given. It is usually shared at the same time that the symbols are conveyed.

91

How many symbols are taught ?

At the Second Degree level three symbols are taught to help create a bridge from the heart of the Reiki channel to the heart of the healee, through which the energy may be drawn. Even at the Second Degree level it is a misnomer to say that you "send" energy because, indeed, this never happens. For this reason you can never invade someone with Reiki. On some level, the other person's body/mind has to be open to receiving the treatment just as in First Degree hands on treatments.

The first symbol is the absent healing symbol which helps the individual create the bridge through which another can draw the energy. The second symbol, often called the mental symbol, is used to help eliminate the mental blocks which cause disease and stress in the first place. The third symbol enables the healee to draw a more amplified version of Reiki as needed, according to the circumstances.

The three Second Degree symbols are never to be taught outside of a class or printed in a book (although some ignorant and spiritually immature people have done so for their own foolish reasons).

~ *92* ~

How long is a Second Degree class?

Mrs. Takata, the woman most responsible for promulgating Reiki in America, often taught Second Degree in only four or five hours. Although she always stressed the necessity for longer First Degree classes so that beginners left fully assured of their ability to convey Reiki, Second Degree with her was short and to the point. It was given only to students who had fully integrated First Degree. Essentially, she gave the Second Degree attunement, taught the three symbols and conveyed the ways and means for sharing distant treatments.

My own classes are set in three approximately four hour segments. In the first segment, I give the attunement and symbols. In the second and third segment I like to share some of the ways I have used Second Degree for my own spiritual growth and development. I also like to give the participants the opportunity to try out Second Degree in the course of the class itself.

❧ 93 ❧

How does Second Degree Reiki differ from First Degree Reiki?

Whereas the attunements of First Degree tend to focus on amplifying the life force energy of the physical body which also often sets off a lot of physical cleansings, the Second Degree attunement seems to have a more intense effect on the etheric or energy body.

Over the years, I have had a lot of feedback from my students about the heightening of their intuitive abilities. Also, quite a few have mentioned experiencing strong sexual feelings (caused by suppressed sexual energy being released). All of these are symptoms of old energy blocks in the etheric body opening up. Basically, the mental body becomes much more fine tuned and as a result intuition is increased. Some people actually develop greater clairaudience, clairvoyance or clairsentience (kinesthetic ability or sensitivity). This enables us to follow our own inner guidance to a much greater degree.

As healers we increase our ability to sense another's needs. Not only do we feel another's needs through our hands, additional more specific information may begin to come through intuitively as well. At this stage I encourage my students to allow themselves to let go of the specific pattern of treatment they learned in First Degree, and follow any impulses which come through.

In general, a further letting go occurs in Second Degree on an energetic level which increases the individual's awareness. It is important at this point not to get impressed with any newfound abilities (such as psychic abilities which may develop), as this will only set you back in your spiritual growth and development. Second Degree can best be approached as a further tool for waking up, rather than something gained from outside of yourself to boost your power.

❧ 94 ❧

What happens in the twenty-one day cleanse process after Second Degree?

The results of the Second Degree cleanse process vary with each individual. There often are further physical cleansings similar to what can happen during the First Degree cleanse process. Also further emotional clearings take place.

What is most common is the gradual noticing of an increased intuitive awareness. For some it is very sudden and dramatic as certain abilities abruptly open up. For most it is a gradual process as one begins to notice after some time a greater sensitivity to those around them, or enhanced perceptiveness in their daily life.

The bottom line is that no individual ever gets more than she or he can handle. Openings in awareness only occur when a person is ready, when all unconscious fears have been sufficiently dealt with. The practice of Reiki at the Second Degree level will itself remove these fears.

❦ 95 ❦

How can I benefit most from Second Degree?

Second Degree's real benefit is the peace you feel after letting go of all of your old resentments, anger and worry. Most people are initially attracted to Second Degree Reiki because they either want to increase their power and intuitive abilities, or they are interested in learning how to do distant treatments on others.

The greatest gift you can receive from Second Degree, however, is freedom from the old mental blocks and patterns which would otherwise keep you in suffering (the kind of innate power you feel when freed of the ego's chains). The main focus of my Second Degree course is teaching my students how to do distant treatments on themselves. With the tools of Second Degree, you are enabled to go back in time and remove the sting of old traumas or painful memories which may still be affecting you in the present.

In all of the world's ancient shamanic traditions, there have always been practices taught which would help the individual draw together all the fragments of self; all the buried incidents which hold sway over the personality, and keep one from experiencing true freedom. By bringing these incidents into full consciousness, acknowledging their lessons and letting them go, we unburden ourselves of sometimes lifetimes of guilt and false obligation.

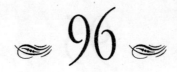

How can I use Second Degree on myself?

Once you have been initiated into Second Degree by a master in the direct lineage of Dr. Usui, and have learned the proper Second Degree symbols, you can create a "bridge" across both time and space to incidents in your past which need healing.

Over a period of years I worked with Reiki, bridging the energy to the time when I was in utero and then worked forward to the present. I worked with each year of my childhood, adolescence, and young adulthood, creating a bridge to myself in the past to which the energy could be drawn.

At first, I worked with incidents I could recall: especially any incident where I was unjustly treated, or out of ignorance by someone, made to feel small or "not good enough". Slowly but surely, through the Reiki energy, old limitations and negative beliefs and doubts I had picked up from others were methodically dealt with.

Although I have always been blessed with a pretty high degree of self confidence and very supportive parents, nevertheless all the societal conditioning which brainwashes you into thinking you are not good enough, you don't know enough, you don't have enough and so forth began to be lifted off my shoulders.

With practice the recollection of events became crystal clear: in each event where someone had tried to make me feel small, I could see their own unconscious inner motivation for doing so: deep unconscious beliefs in their own unworthiness. It became easier to not take people personally and also to not react back unconsciously out of a similar ignorance and insensitivity.

Slowly but surely there was no longer a need to call up the ego to "protect" me as it became apparent there is no separate "other" to be protected from. As most of life's burdens were lifted, a sense of peace began to supplant my earlier self confidence: a sense of peace not dependent on feeling good versus "bad", or happy versus "sad", or even up versus "down" — just plain and simple peace and non-causal joy.

What is the real secret of Second Degree?

Eventually, after using Second Degree for a period of years to recollect and discharge the energy of old stuck patterns, you may discover its secret: that truly there is no time and space to traverse, that they do not exist! At the highest degree of understanding, time and space are actually only concepts which describe how a human being experiences all of life's circumstances in a linear fashion.

It is difficult for the human mind with its attachment to the five senses to comprehend that there is no past, present or future, that in actual fact everything is happening all at once. This is why, for example, the ancient Rishis in India, or Nostradamus in the west, could see into the "future". They simply had vast peripheral or panoramic vision.

After a period of years, as you dissolve a lot of *attachments* to your beliefs and behavior patterns, as you get in touch with the non-causal joy which lies beneath all of your surface patterns, a major shift can take place. At a certain point, the entire illusion of time and space can fall away and leave you with a direct experience of Self. As each of the seeming memories of the past are recalled and brought into the present, the past literally shrinks until there is only one vast and limitless present.

In that moment, there is actually no "you" or ego left, for the experiencer simply disappears. Later, the memory or ego of the body/mind may remember that "something" happened and tend to claim the experience, but from then on everything is not quite the same. The sense of the unlimitedness of who you truly are, can then call you into the non-causal freedom that is now able to express itself through you.

⮬ 98 ⮬

How can I use Second Degree to do distant treatments on others?

After receiving the Second Degree attunement from a qualified Reiki master and learning the three symbols, you will be taught how to create a bridge from your heart to the heart of another, across which the energy can be drawn. Just as with First Degree, it is important that the person ask for a treatment.

However, you cannot "invade" someone with Second Degree Reiki because even at this level the energy is *drawn*, not sent or projected. In cases, for example, when someone is in a coma and is therefore in no position to ask for a treatment, you can always create a bridge, begin the treatment, and notice if the person actually starts to draw energy. You will feel if they are drawing or not. If they draw energy then you can continue the treatment. If not, you simply cease the treatment.

Why are the symbols and the descriptions of the attunements not to be published in a book? Are they secret?

Attunements can only be properly given by a person who has used Reiki for a considerable amount of time (i.e. usually several years), and has fully imbibed the essence of Reiki so that it then can be passed on. Although there is a specific form or ritual to the attunements or empowerments, the form remains worthless, if given by someone without any energy or experience behind them; if they have not fully embodied Reiki. It is much the same with the symbols for Second and Third Degree.

Some very ignorant people have begun publishing the Reiki symbols and describing the attunement process in books (most of these descriptions, by the way are inaccurate). They seem to have the idea that the general populace is ready to learn from a book, what must actually be conveyed *directly* from master to student.

You cannot receive Reiki empowerments through a book, by correspondence, or over the internet. The attunements must be given directly from one human being to another, and they can only be given by someone who is fully *qualified* and *experienced*.

Second Degree Symbols are only meant to be given to First Degree students who have a lot of experience under their belt and have developed confidence and trust in the efficacy of Reiki. A minimum of three to six months of experience at the First Degree level is important to fully gain the benefit of Second Degree.

Also, the Second Degree symbols will not work if you have not been attuned at the Second Degree level by someone who carries the essence. The point of not printing the symbols in a book or elsewhere is threefold: First of all, you don't give a nursery school student high school level information. As Jesus said: "You don't cast pearls before swines." They won't be able to absorb it. Secondly, Reiki can never be "known" or understood intellectually. It can only be *experienced*. You can indeed talk about it, but really only to relieve the mind's doubts. Head knowledge does not help you share better treatments or raise your life force energy. It often only creates more confusion if not laid out simply. Thirdly and most important of which most of the people who have printed the symbols are unaware: Although there have been a few power monger types in Reiki, as in all things human, for the most part the Reiki symbols and attunement procedures have not been held back or kept secret from anyone because an alleged "Reiki elite" wanted it so for the sake of their own power. It is purposely only shared with properly prepared students who are ready to use the symbols with the same intention as every practitioner in the long Reiki tradition.

It is important to understand that most human beings are entirely unaware of the power of the human mind. For example, in my *Core Abundance Seminar*, I always caution my students not to share their goals with others until the foundation is laid and they are well on their way to actually manifesting them in physical reality. If you share your ideas prematurely, others most often will (unconsciously) think: "Oh, so and so, he or she will never accomplish that goal or that project!", and will actually dissipate the energy of your project.

The average human mind, due to false conditioning, dwells often on the negative polarity, and exposing your ideas to such negativity will only dissipate the energy of your project. You also want to keep the energy *condensed* so it will support you. I encourage them only to share their ideas with the few people around them who have a positive mindset.

The same is pertinent for Reiki. It has always been important to only share the symbols with people who are ready to use them with the proper intention. To show them to an unknowledgeable, doubting person (let alone a huge public) who might think: "What is this gobbledey gook?" would only dissipate their energy. Fortunately today, however, Reiki is so widespread, ignorant negativity will probably no longer act to dissipate their power. There are just too many Reiki practitioners, all with the same positive intention.

Still, the proper attunements which are received directly from a fully qualified master are the only way, Second and Third Degree symbols or attunements have any efficacy. Thus, what is the point of publishing them except sheer greed, ignorance, or the naive presupposition that you can save the world with them, as if the world needed saving.

The world may indeed appear imperfect in your eyes, and doubtless there is much strife. However, the approach to relieving this pain is to abstain from meddling in the affairs of others (except for emergencies when your intervention is clearly called for), but rather invoke the absolute perfection inherent in all being and beings.

You do not want to subject the symbols and attunements to the distortion of the outside world. You want to keep them hidden so that they can silently and miraculously transform the world into what it essentially already IS: Awareness, Consciousness, Bliss.

❧ 100 ❧

Does Second Degree amplify my power?

What Second Degree actually does, is increase your body/mind's life force energy. Through the Second Degree attunement, the vibratory frequency of the physical body, with a special emphasis on the energy body, is boosted. As a result, you are able to channel at a higher (or lighter) frequency. Essentially, what you experience is a "de-densification", as more dense energy is let go of. This may make you feel more "powerful" simply because you are now much more in touch with what had always been available, but that you previously couldn't access due to your having been stuck in beliefs, judgments and limitations.

THIRD DEGREE BASICS

❧ 101 ❧

What is Third Degree?

Third Degree is effectively the teaching level of the Usui Method Of Natural Healing (*Usui Shiki Ryoho*). At the Third Degree level, you learn one more symbol and receive the Third Degree attunement. You also learn how to convey the First and Second Degree attunements and how to properly organize and teach Reiki classes.

The Third Degree training takes at least about a year in itself and should only be considered after a teacher and student have known each other through working together for a minimum of one full year. This way, the teacher can act as a proper mirror for whatever the student needs to learn, because a bond of trust has been well established.

102

Do I need Third Degree to increase my power?

Much like Second Degree, Third Degree is more about fine tuning your life force energy (and not so much about amplifying your power). Unfortunately, what most people still don't understand, is that while First and Second Degree are about empowering you by putting you in touch with the direct connection you've always had, but previously never realized, with all the energy there is, Third Degree is about dropping your desire and need for power. In other words, Third Degree is about dropping the ego's drive to be "better" or more "powerful", and to finally realizing that *You Are* Reiki Itself (so that all sense of separation falls off like a garment that has been outgrown).

If Second Degree is used to its greatest advantage for several years, its benefit will make Third Degree a moot point in terms of further "empowerment".

103

What should be my motivation for Third Degree?

The only reason for Third Degree is the intense desire to teach Reiki. If your idea is to "save the world", I would suggest first doing some deep self inquiry to help put your missionary zeal in perspective. It is important to get in touch with what is ultimately real, so that you can discover there is no world (outside of yourself) to be saved. It is essential before teaching anything to first acknowledge your real motives (especially the subconscious ones) for wanting to teach. Once they are brought to full awareness, they can no longer control you, and you won't tend to project them on others.

For example, some people teach in order to gain respect and love from their students, to control others, to boost their ego and so forth. All of which are not a serious problem, as long you are aware of them and can at least admit these tendencies to yourself and others. If this is the case, you will have half a chance to not fall for them (and if you do fall for them occasionally, you'll snap out of it quickly). Naturally, most people who desire to teach also have altruistic ideas about teaching, but to be a teacher who can actually help benefit students, you need to be aware of all the shadow aspects of your personality.

The whole point of teaching from the standpoint of the teacher's own growth, is to empty the proverbial cup.... it is to realize that truly there is no teacher and no student: there are only two human beings sharing the joy of remembering who they truly are. If this is your motivation, you'll be a fantastic teacher!

〜 104 〜

How long should I practice Reiki before considering Third Degree?

Since Third Degree is a training for teachers, it is necessary that you be equipped with a full knowledge of First and Second Degree through direct personal experience. It takes three to six months of using First Degree just to get a basic understanding of how Reiki can affect different people in different situations. This experience can only be gained by treating many different ailments. Furthermore, you need to imbibe the changes in yourself (which result from self treatments and from treating others).

Second Degree provides a tool for releasing the charge of old, unnecessary mental and emotional patterns. Extensive work at this level is needed to not only disengage from your own ego identification, but also to learn about the various ways Second Degree can support others. A group of the original masters trained by Takata, plus their first few trainees from the early eighties have all come to the conclusion that three years of experience is what is really necessary to be fully prepared to teach Reiki.

I myself tried teaching masters after only one year of experience. I found the results to be far from beneficial. Much of an individual's unfinished business seems to come to the surface, and then it is just taken out or projected on their students. Although three years of experience is my requirement or guideline, sometimes even that is not enough time. For some individuals more time is needed in preparation for teaching.

Furthermore, not everyone asking for Third Degree may deep down, really want or need the teaching level of Reiki, but may make the request because subconsciously the need is for something else. In such cases, through empathic resonance, it is up to the teacher to uncover the real need and help the student by pointing out a way to fulfillment.

❧ 105 ❧

Is there such a thing as separate 3A and 3B master levels, or a special training for grand masters?

Third Degree is always to be taught as a whole and not subdivided. There may be steps and stages in the teaching, but giving only the attunement to Third Degree as an end in itself and calling it "3A", is not recommended. This practice was started by one of the original Reiki masters who, as I understand it, went very much against her teacher's, (Mrs. Takata's) wishes.

This particular master decided that she would give the Third Degree attunement and symbol to people who wanted to use Reiki only for their spiritual growth and not to teach. For people who wanted to teach Reiki, she would convey how to transmit the First and Second Degree attunements, but she withheld the process of how to conduct the empowerment into Third Degree. This she called "3B".

As I've already pointed out many times, Third Degree is not about amplifying your power, rather it is about *dropping* your power trip, your attachment to the belief that you need to be powerful or have a powerful personality. Therefore, "3A" is redundant, because you can only gain the real benefit (and by this I mean spiritual benefit) of Third Degree when you actually start teaching, and in the process begin to "empty your cup". Through teaching you actually put yourself on the line and your ego under the scrutiny of your students. In this way, your students will also become your teachers which is a very healthy reality check. Basic common sense should also tell you that there can be no "half masters". Unfortunately, two of my own master students who had been influenced by this renegade master, have contributed to the resulting confusion caused by this practice.

Courses in "grand mastership" are the height of absurdity because in Reiki there are no grand masters, and neither are there in any other truly spiritual practice. Hierarchical distinctions such as "grand Mastership" always appear on the horizon when a live spiritual tradition is about to lose its freshness and begins to turn into a quasi political religious organization. This can never be the purpose of Reiki which essentially is an immediate access to the health and wholeness that you always already are. An ongoing experience of such immediacy would only be compromised, if subjected to the weight of dead hierarchies.

The lack of any hierarchies, on the other hand, places a lot of responsibility into the hands of each and every Reiki practitioner. Since there is no one above you to keep your ego in line, you have to open to intrinsic awareness or the Energy Itself to guide your daily actions.

106

Can Third Degree be taught like a seminar or a class ?

No, absolutely not! Third Degree is a one to one proposition. Occasionally, I have worked with two or three people simultaneously for parts of their training, but it is necessary to give a Third Degree student a lot of personal attention.

The master/student relationship at Third Degree level is for a lifetime. It is also necessary that your master gets to know you for at least one year before actually starting with the training so that he or she can address your particular needs.

These fly by night "instant" Third Degree seminars are simply just money making propositions. The modern tendency to less and less direct human contact and interaction does not suffice with Reiki.

107

What are the requirements and preparation for Third Degree ?

There needs to be a minimum of three years experience as a Reiki practitioner. This translates to daily self treatment, plus plenty of experience working on many different people, preferably in your own Reiki clinic.

My own Third Degree students are required to have worked with me for at least one year, preferably organizing a few classes for me in order to learn organizational skills. Most of all, this time together allows us to develop a bond of trust, so that the student can really receive what I have to teach. I may also suggest other seminars or reading according to each student's ability and to broaden their scope so they are better prepared for their own students' questions later on. Another thing I suggest is that my student audit other teachers' classes just to get a feeling for different styles of teaching.

This initial relationship also enables me to get to know my student and all of his or her patterns and quirks so I can better point them out. To further this end, I also require that my master students take the *Core Empowerment Training* at least three times to fully drop their attachment to teaching, so that paradoxically they become better teachers. Any kind of self-assessment work or direct self inquiry can also help to this end.

Thus the main requirements for Third Degree are first, a strong desire to teach. Secondly, there are the mechanical requirements of three years' experience, a broadening of scope, and a deepening of self-knowledge (to know and help others you must first know and help yourself). Thirdly, there is an exchange of energy which needs to be completed beforehand.

The exchange of energy needs to be completed before the training begins and the attunement is given, as it is wise not to become your student's "banker". Also, the exchange of energy needs to be in keeping with the student's capability, yet also needs to stretch their limits to a large degree to show that they are indeed in earnest. This is helpful, because it is necessary for a student to be really sincere, to actually benefit from Third Degree. Thus for a multimillionaire student for

whom money means nothing, you would have to become
creative. You might have to come up with some type of service
they could give to others, or some other way they actually
share their time which is often more precious to them than
money. Although nowadays money is most commonly used
as an exchange of energy, I have sometimes retained services
or artwork from my students.

By much trial and error, I have learned to always write
a contract with my Third Degree students so that everything
is up front and later there are no misunderstandings.

$$108$$

How is Third Degree taught?

Third Degree has to be molded differently according to each
student's needs. After all the preliminary preparation is dealt
with and the exchange of energy is complete, the student and
I choose a time to begin the first portion of the training. This
usually consists of a number of days together when the Third
Degree attunement and symbol are conveyed, and the process
of how to go about giving the First Degree attunements is
taught and then practiced. Also given are other beneficial
practices which help the student absorb the teaching. At the
end of this first portion of the training, we usually teach a
First Degree class together.

It is then up to the master student to organize and teach
a number of First Degree classes for about three to six months,
after which time I then teach the process of how to convey

the Second Degree attunements. This portion of the training is than completed with a Second Degree class that we teach together. From then on, the master student can begin to teach Second Degree.

It is only after a lengthy period of teaching both First and Second Degree classes that the process for conveying the Third Degree attunement is taught. Part of the contract for Third Degree is that the master student promises not to teach another Third Degree master student him- or herself for at least three years, and to teach at least twenty First Degree classes with a minimum of twelve students (forty classes with five or six students will do) and at least fifteen to twenty Second Degree classes. In order to convey the mastership properly you have to be a well schooled, very experienced teacher yourself. Beware of so-called masters who have received mastership after only six months experience, not to mention some of the fly by night produced in less than a month.

My advice for potential master students is to fully query your potential teacher. If you are looking for the cheapest master on the block, you are probably not ready for Third Degree. To get the most benefit of Third Degree find someone who is really willing to take time with you and stretch you to your limit. Find someone who doesn't make you feel small or less than he or she, but honors you and shows you love and respect. Definitely, avoid anyone who is attempting to elicit fear in you in any form. In Indian traditions a spiritual teacher is sometimes referred to as "friend in wholesomeness" (kalyanamitra). If this is your desire, find your wholesome friend so that you may find peace.

THE FULL BODY TREATMENT AND ITS EFFECT ON THE ENDOCRINE SYSTEM

Traditional Reiki emphasizes the importance of first treating the whole body by utilizing hand positions which cover all the major organs and the key endocrine glands, and only after that completing the treatment on specific trouble spots. The life force needs to be raised throughout the entire body in order to summon the self healing powers inherent in our physical structure. All of the glands of the endocrine system work together to keep the body in perfect balance. By enhancing and energizing the endocrine glands, much that is out of order will naturally begin to synchronize, and once having been mobilized, the innate self healing power of the body can be brought to bear on the area affected by a specific ailment.

As the body is a whole in which any part or level of structural organization is interrelated and interacts with any other part or level of structural organization, it logically follows that we do have to treat the whole in order to balance and heal the part. Naturally, the opposite is also true: whenever we let just one area of the body draw Reiki, the whole body also benefits indirectly because no matter where you lay on your hands, the energy is always drawn to where it is most needed.

The spontaneous laying on of hands, wherever we feel drawn to do so, is usually sufficient for the general maintenance of life force energy in your body. However, for treating specific imbalances or ailments, this approach may not provide an energy boost strong enough to make a difference. From this it logically follows that, full body treatments are required.

In order to understand what is involved, it is helpful to review which areas and systems of the body are covered by the traditional hand positions during a full body Reiki treatment: By covering the body from head to toe, we inadvertently treat the nervous system, the bones of the skeleton and the muscles. We also cover many parts of the skin. Furthermore, particular attention is given to the organs, which include the cardiovascular, lymphatic, digestive, urinary, respiratory, and reproductive systems. Throughout the process we also put extra attention on the endocrine system.

Thus a full body treatment with Reiki enhances the interplay of the eleven major functional systems of our bodies. For example, through strengthening the circulatory system by letting the heart draw Universal Life Force Energy, we automatically strengthen the respiratory system, because more oxygen-laden blood can be distributed, and more "used" blood filled with carbon dioxide can be delivered for disposal by the lungs. Or, by letting the pancreas draw Reiki you simultaneously raise the life force energy in your digestive and endocrine systems because the pancreas happens to be part of both of them.

There are countless similarly important connections. They are far too numerous, to mention all of them. However, it might be helpful for your Reiki practice, to learn more about this miraculous living continuum of the human body, the many interactions among its systems and their mysterious, life sustaining synergy. Further reading is highly suggested. There are many excellent and beautifully illustrated books available about the workings of the human body. Pick one up at your local library and start investigating on your own. It is helpful to read with your heart as well as with your mind. You can absorb and analyze the factual information, but also allow yourself to be touched by the beauty and incredible complexity of what we call a human body, your very own vehicle for experiencing this dimension. Also know that whatever you learn during your investigation is just a fraction of what is there, because the more factual knowledge you acquire, the more you realize how much more there is, that you don't know. Any increase in factual knowledge always automatically increases our ignorance regarding new levels of factual knowledge that are implied by the bits and pieces that have just been uncovered. Thus it is that we must honor the intuition (the truth) of the moment in addition to our factual knowledge. It is much like the wisdom of the ancients which recognizes that we can never really *know* anything, that we can only *experience* it.

Your newly found knowledge will eventually fine tune the direct sensations and feelings which tend to come up during a treatment and greatly deepen your understanding of Reiki. Clarity and precision will begin to replace vague and cloudy impressions. Of course, feeling directly what is happening in the moment remains the most important factor in your practice. However, combined with clear insights into the workings of the human body, the ability to feel will help you to communicate your intuitions and perceptions to yourself and others in a much clearer fashion, which in turn will empower you to be of greater assistance.

Reiki always acts in the same manner: it raises the life force energy and calms the mind. In other words, it simultaneously hones your energy *and* creates balance. The more the whole body is suffused with it, the higher and more balanced will its vibratory frequency become, i.e. it becomes less susceptible to disharmony, degeneration and atrophy. A key to dispersing Reiki throughout the entire body is to place special emphasis on the endocrine system.

Together with the interlocking nervous system, we could call the endocrine system the main regulator of the body. It consists of several glands of internal secretion that yield the hormones which govern our growth from childhood to adulthood and control our sexual development. It is also closely connected to and interacts with the immune system, which protects us against disease. These systems and the hormones they produce, direct virtually every bodily function, from breathing to digestion, to reproduction, to fending off disease. They enable the body to deal with heat, cold, stress and starvation, and help it to protect itself against dehydration, infection, trauma and bleeding. They also control the volume of the body fluids and their chemical composition and balance.

The endocrine or ductless glands are: The hypothalamus, the pineal gland, the pituitary gland, the thyroid and parathyroid glands, the thymus, the adrenal cortex and medulla, the pancreas, the ovaries (in women), and the testes (in men). They produce most of the hormones which control a multitude of functions and rhythms of the body. However, several other organs also secrete hormones. The stomach, liver, intestines, kidneys, and heart all contain clusters of cells which emit hormones into the bloodstream, and thus become part of the endocrine system (although they themselves are not endocrine glands in the strictest sense of the word).

It would go beyond the scope of this short essay to fully describe the entire workings of the endocrine system. Two examples will suffice to illustrate the case in point. They may give you a better idea of its importance and motivate you to learn more about it and also to direct more Reiki to the endocrine glands.

Since ancient times, the pineal gland was believed to be important, although in most historical periods and especially in western culture little was known about this tiny structure in the shape of a pine cone (hence its name). To the French philosopher and mathematician René Descartes, the pineal gland was the mysterious place where "mind and body meet". Today, our knowledge is more specific: We now realize that in one sense, the pineal gland serves as an internal clock, regulating the circadian rhythms of the body, i.e. it makes sure that we stay attuned to daily and seasonal changes. It enables us to live in synchronicity with nature by regulating the body's wake/sleep cycle in accordance with the earth's cycle of day and night.

However, regulating the body's wake/sleep cycle is just one of the many tasks taken up by the pineal gland. Its even more crucial function, according to recent research, is akin to a lifelong internal timer. In this capacity, the pineal gland performs the task of the body's aging clock which controls the aging process by releasing the hormone melatonin, which then transmits information to other systems in the body telling them how and when to age. In other words, our physical bodies grow up, mature and degenerate because the melatonin level in the pineal gland instructs them to. The adult peak level for melatonin is at around age twenty, but by age sixty we have only half of the melatonin available with further dramatic slips which continue, and, of course, accelerate the process of degeneration even further into what we usually call "old age".

The question then is, does this new found knowledge about

the function of the pineal gland give us a clue about a potential slowing down of the aging process? It very well may. Some go even so far as to suggest that by treating the body with hormonal supplements, we are actually able not only to stop but to reverse the aging process. In the context of Reiki another question then arises, if we can indeed reset the aging clock in the pineal gland by supplementing the body with melatonin, would regular Reiki treatments on this very gland achieve the same goal of maintaining life in a strong and healthy body even in old age so that you would eventually die without being subjected to the typical ailments of degeneration? Historical accounts from Taoist and Tantric masters and adepts who have channeled and applied Universal Life Force Energy in their practice strongly suggest this as a fact.

However at this point we have to acknowledge how truly groundbreaking Mrs. Takata's focus on the endocrine system really was during her lifetime, because most of the information on the endocrine system available now had not yet come out in 1980 when she passed away. Actually, until the late seventies most researchers still believed that every gland and every organ system performed solo, wholly independent of other glands and organ systems. It was proved only later, that the glands of the endocrine system are in constant contact and interaction with the cells of the immune system. Still later it was found that there must be some governing agency in the body that was designed to coordinate the exchange of information to carry out the task of executing all of these functions.

The pineal gland is this governing agency. As long as it produces sufficient amounts of melatonin, our immune system will be vigorous and we will be endowed with high levels of lymphocytes (which create antibodies and suppress unwanted invaders). The level of the thyroid hormone in the body will also stay high to provide for a higher level of energy.

It is also very likely that health will be maintained into the very last days of our life and that age related cancer will not occur, which is why regular Reiki on the pineal gland will promote much more than simple longevity. It will also greatly enhance the quality of life.

The most important quality of Reiki is that it releases tension and stress. According Dr. Usui's own statement on the subject, Reiki was designed "to calm the mind and raise the life force energy". In this way it exerts a strong healing influence on the immune system and may prevent much stress induced illness.

Stress causes a great deal of damage to the immune system. There are many studies available on the subject which prove beyond any doubt that stress induced illness is indeed happening and that stress is at least a contributing factor in many diseases, and very often actually triggers it. Stress takes many forms in a human being, for example: conflicts at home, work related anxieties, sleep deprivation, the typical modern day over stimulation of the senses combined with a simultaneous lack of physical exercise, taking care of chronically ill family members and so forth. Immune suppression and stress can therefore be regarded as synonymous.

In other words, the more stress there is in your life, and the more you *identify* with this stress by perceiving yourself as its victim, the more suppressed your immune system will be, and the more you are likely to suffer from stress induced illness; particularly if your personal response to outside stress is to create even more inner strife and stress.

Basically, stress awakens the flight-or-fight response. It stimulates the sympathetic nervous system and suppresses the parasympathetic nervous system, which is responsible for bodily functions in times of rest, relaxation, meditation and deep sleep. It shouldn't come as a surprise to us that the immune system functions better when the parasympathetic nervous system kicks in and takes over. On the other hand, when the body is preparing to fight or flee, dealing with an invading micro-organism is definitely not its top priority.

The secretion of stress induced adrenal gland hormones then inhibit white blood cell function and lower the production of lymphocytes. Continued subjection to external and reactive internal stress may even cause the thymus gland to shrink (the thymus gland being the master gland of the immune system). A significant reduction in immune system activity is both the immediate and long term result. The message is clear and simple: stress really does damage immune function.

Regular Reiki on all the glands of the endocrine system, particularly on the area of the thymus gland will counteract this trend, and eventually lead to an alteration in the neurotransmitters in your brain because you will open gradually to more positive thoughts such as love, compassion, peace, personal courage, commitment and self actualization.

As we all know from our own experience: negative thoughts make us feel down (in other words: suppress the immune system). Positive thoughts on the other hand, when palpably felt, stimulate the immune system. More studies on the effect of positive thoughts on the neurotransmitters in our brain are coming out every year, changing the focus of research from disease producing mechanisms to health engendering mechanisms (which in itself is a very healthy change).

Through actively supporting neuro-immune modulation in the course of a treatment or self treatment (by strengthening the interaction between the endocrine and immune systems of the body and their link to the brain), Reiki is quickly becoming a gentle form of mind/body medicine. Regular application of Universal Life Force Energy will have a spill-over effect on pretty much every area of your life.

Provided you do Reiki more than just once in a while, it is very likely that the four primary areas of expression will be affected by the regular application of Universal Life Force Energy. As a result, in your daily existence, you will find a new and mutually enhancing and nurturing balance. You will intuitively know, how long it is appropriate to work, when you need to play, when and where it is appropriate to open yourself to love, and when and how to express your deep faith in Self.

WHY REIKI?

Naturopathy suggests that there is really only one healing power in existence, and that is Nature Herself. In Reiki we call this healing power Universal Life Force Energy, which includes but goes far beyond the ordinary inherent restorative power of the body to battle and vanquish disease. As an added benefit it touches upon and includes the potential for complete self realization in moment to moment awareness. Since in Reiki we directly work with energy, Reiki itself is considered a form of energy medicine.

Like other forms of natural healing, Reiki also stresses the importance of health maintenance and disease prevention which is a much cheaper and more effective approach to well being than the common focus on curing manifest diseases. Toward the end of his life even Louis Pasteur, the father of the allopathic "war on germs", conceded as much. Throughout his professional life Pasteur had fought for the acceptance of his theory that each disease is produced by a different infectious micro-organism. On the grounds of this view, he had battled his fellow French scientist Claude Bernard who held forth that the *susceptibility* of an individual to these infectious micro-organisms was actually more important than the micro-organisms themselves. Although Pasteur eventually convinced pretty much everyone of the correctness of his views, he himself was forthright enough to admit that he had been wrong, because shortly before his death he himself stated: "Bernard was right. The pathogen is nothing. The terrain is everything." Which means that even Pasteur finally came to see that the state of a person's internal environment contributes much more to their tendency to manifest a disease than the infecting organisms or pathogens themselves.

Although antibiotics are extremely helpful in cases of serious infections and life threatening diseases, the general obsession with the killing of invading micro-organisms (rather than strengthening and supporting the immune system through maintaining good health and psychophysical balance) automatically leads to many instances of improper usage. The misuse of these powerful antibiotic agents, such as prescribing them thoughtlessly for a common cold or flu has become rampant in many countries in the world. Through the misuse which has happened over the past forty to fifty years, we are in danger of losing their curative powers, because more and more micro-organisms are becoming resistant to antibiotics. According to many experts we are already too close for comfort to a "post-antibiotic era" in which numerous infectious diseases will once again become as incurable as they were in the "pre-antibiotic era".

This is why the nature cure or Reiki approach to maintaining good health are crucial not only to individual well-being but to a healthier health care system in general. The need for a healthier approach to health care is precisely why many medical doctors on the cutting edge are looking for a more holistic paradigm. Although still in the minority, their numbers are increasing steadily. With insurance companies, in the framework of so-called "managed care", now dictating the types of treatments physicians can use, they are becoming painfully aware of the disruptive and outright destructive ways the present day health care industry is destroying actual health care.

Indeed, much is afoul with the still predominant paradigm which views good health only as a physical state which reflects the absence of any manifest disease. We basically can no longer afford for an approach which is about to bankrupt us both physically and fiscally. We have no other choice but to support techniques and therapies which will teach us how to stay well. The following figures speak for themselves:

According to the *American Journal of Health Promotion*, we spent $ US 1 Trillion ($ 1,000,000,000,000!!) on the treatment of diseases in the United States of America in 1994, and the expenditures for so-called "health care" have skyrocketed by a whopping 300% in the last 15 years alone. Disease is obviously a very lucrative business! At present, the treatment of diseases consumes more than 15% of the gross national product of this country and continues to rise at twice the rate of inflation (whereas in 1930 it only consumed 1.9%!)

Obviously, something went terribly wrong because, not only do Americans spend more money than ever on the treatment of disease, they are on the average also less healthy than they were when they spent only ten percent of what they are spending now! What happened?

The reasons are many, but they can pretty much be summarized in two factors: In the thirties big money interests started to push for legislation which severely restricted (and to a larger extent today continues to restrict and even terrorize) complementary approaches to health care. At the same time, through different foundations under the guise of charity, the drug industry began to pour big dollars into medical schools, gradually seeing to it that curriculums were changed in a way that would profit them down the road. In short, disease began to have commercial value, and health went down the tubes.

In the sixties and seventies, the government stepped in

and made the situation even worse. Federal and state subsidies inflated the number of graduating medical doctors, doubling the rate between 1965 and 1980 so that in 1992 there were 245 doctors per 100,000 Americans, whereas in 1970 the ratio had been 151 doctors per 100,000 Americans (a staggering increase of 62%!). Furthermore, most of the new doctors are not general practitioners but specialists who tend to prescribe and utilize the most expensive procedures. This might at first seem to be a tribute to modern health care. Wouldn't the fact that there are more specialists at hand and ready to help, imply that Americans are medically better cared for than ever before?

Not so, concludes a study conducted in the late eighties which found that a geographical area with 4.5 surgeons per 10,000 population had 940 operations whereas an area with 2.5 surgeons for the same amount of people experienced only 590 operations in the same stretch of time. To put it bluntly: If you double the amount of surgeons you end up with double the amount of surgeries! The question then is: are they all necessary?

You bet they aren't, says another study published in the *Journal of the American Medical Association* on 168 patients who were either scheduled or counseled to undergo coronary artery bypass surgery. The study found the proposed surgery in 80% of the cases either unnecessary or inappropriate. In other words: Less than 34 of 168 patients set for surgery really needed surgery!

Many things are wrong with our view of the treatment of disease and with the health care industry which is in the business of making money off diseases (not off health and well-being), it is no wonder that we no longer hear much reference to healing as an art. The way the game is set up right now, it is virtually impossible to shift the interest of the "health" care industry to health because too much money is made from disease. This doesn't imply a sinister conspiracy by individual health care practitioners like doctors and nurses. Most try their best according to their training and the information that is available to them. Quite a few would be shocked if they knew that the costs of preventable prescription drug related diseases and deaths amounted to $ US 77 billion in the early nineties, and are most likely considerably higher now!

Despite the trillion dollars spent on the treatment of diseases (or is it *because* that much money was spent ?) almost half of all working Americans are in ill health or suffer from a chronic disease (such as arthritis, high blood pressure, diabetes and so forth). Please take note, that this figure only takes into account people in their prime who are a part of the work force. The numbers for the elderly are far worse, virtually all of whom are afflicted by one or more chronic and/ or degenerative conditions!

All the above data, of which there is much more on iatrogenic (physician caused disease), clearly suggest that a change in outlook is called for. A shift in focus is needed from treating diseases to maintaining health. Because of its openness and versatility, as well as its emphasis on prevention, Reiki is an integral part of the newly emerging care for the whole person. According to this new paradigm, health is seen as a state of optimal physical, mental, emotional and spiritual well-being or, to use another common phrase: as total wellness. Total wellness is also both the nature and the aim of Universal Life Force Energy.

The pending shift in the health care paradigm, by the way,

does not mean that we have to discard anything which was gained over many years or even generations of dedicated medical research. There will always be a place for state of the art modern allopathic forms of treatment, simply because there are countless instances when they are a real blessing and save lives, as for example in trauma surgery.

Nowhere in this book or in this short essay did we infer that Reiki should replace all other forms of medical intervention. Reiki is in itself a complete form of energy medicine, but it is not a cure all, and neither is any other particular form of medicine. Each discipline offers its own wonderful tools to promote the healing process. When skillfully combined, different forms of medicine can help cure many conditions. The greatest benefit of any healing art, is in strengthening the mind/body continuum to better withstand disease.

In countries such as India or China, which still have a living tradition of age old disease prevention and holistic health care like Ayurveda or Acupuncture, many allopaths are beginning to see the light and adopt some of the ancient tried and true practices. They are well advised to keep their old systems in place, and only supplement them with modern western allopathy in areas where the old system does not provide for the same advanced level of care. The figures and trends discussed above clearly demonstrate the need for caution concerning any wholesale dismissal of long proven, age old healing arts with a several thousand year success rate. The ongoing sneaky attempt and partial success by multinational pharmaceutical companies to patent common ancient Ayurvedic remedies such as neem and turmeric (most often to keep them *out* of circulation) should act as a major wake up call to people everywhere who value freedom of choice in caring for their own bodies.

THE REIKI DECLARATION OF INDEPENDENCE

In Caring For Your Own And/Or Another's Health

The practice of Reiki amounts to a powerful personal *Declaration of Independence* from the crutches and clutches of the typical passive consumer approach to well-being, still predominant in this country and throughout the westernized world. With Reiki you are, in effect, boldly stating that you are (or at least have direct access to) the very energy, you yourself and the entire cosmos are made of, and that, furthermore, this energy will henceforth be the main source of your health and happiness.

This implies that you find certain truths self evident, first and foremost among which is the insight that, in order to be well, you have to be in charge of all matters regarding your own physical, psychological, and spiritual well being. You cease to delegate this power to someone else. Although you will remain perfectly open and available to listen to pertinent advice, you reserve the right to act on *any* outside information according to your own deliberations (and after getting at least a second or even third opinion from whichever source of your own choice). You decide. You don't let so-called specialists decide for you.

In other words you empower yourself to stand up for the truth that you, like all women and men everywhere throughout the whole world, are created equal by the God Force and that you therefore have certain un-alienable rights like the right to life, liberty and the *pursuit* of your own happiness.

You fully understand that Natural Law cannot grant you the right to happiness, for the simple reason that such a "right" would take away your power. Anyone who claims to give you the right to something beyond the basic rights such as life, liberty and the pursuit of happiness, in effect is attempting to grant you a privilege. The problem with privileges (which are similar to inferior civil rights as compared to natural, *un-a-lien-*able rights) is that they can be revoked by the very people who appoint themselves to grant them. A right based on Natural Law, on the other hand, is not as shaky as a mere privilege. It can never be taken away from you because it is your birthright as a free human being.

The right to the pursuit of your own happiness includes the right to choose how you want to take care of your own health. In other words: you have the right to choose the method of treatment you prefer. If there is any outside interference in this process, then your natural right to the pursuit of your own happiness has been ursurped and taken away from you. Furthermore, with the practice of Reiki you make a bold statement that you are well equipped to maintain your own health.

You acknowledge that the body is not a machine separate from all other bodies and all of creation, but that it partakes in the same energies that everything is fundamentally made of. You know that in order to heal the body you will have to address the wholeness that you are, or if you are working as a health care professional, that you will always have to address the whole patient (client). You are aware that your focus has to shift from the elimination of disease to achieving and maintaining good health. You are not so much preoccupied any longer with treating symptoms but rather graduate to the higher level of treating the underlying physical, emotional, socio-economic and spiritual causes. You don't any longer buy into the lie that you have to be emotinally shut down and removed (like a psychotherapist or doctor who believes that he has to protect himself from his patient's feelings) in order to heal yourself and others; instead you know that a little bit of empathy goes a long way, and that directly feeling your own and/or another's pain (which helps release it and allow it to flow through) is actually the first step to removing the causes of this very same pain. In other words, you stop focusing solely on objective information (charts, statistics, test results, book knowledge) to the exclusion of all other sources of information; rather, in addition you take into account how you yourself or your patient (client) are feeling.

Treating yourself and others with Universal Life Force Energy, you do not become dogmatic in any way. According to the writings found in his rediscovered diaries, Dr. Usui, the founder of modern day Reiki, was open to applying whatever means were called for in a given situation. He used Universal Life Force Energy, meditations and ceremonies, western allopathic remedies, common sense counseling, together with Japanese and Chinese naturopathic herbal formulas and more refined gem based elixirs.

In the same spirit of eclecticism, you would probably choose to get shots when bitten by a rabid dog, and you will also gladly avail yourself of the full array of trauma surgery if you become a victim of a bad car accident. However, for example, you would not give your doctor blanket permission to surgically remove your spleen solely as a preventive measure (because spleens, it has been observed, are in danger of rupturing in car accidents). If there is no indication of internal bleeding, you might rather opt for staying in the intensive care unit for a few days to wait and see, if the spleen has indeed been damaged. If not, you could decline surgery.

The most important effect of Reiki is in prevention and in changing your outlook and attitude from dependency and uninformed consumerism to the spirit of sovereignty and self reliance. If you treat yourself with Universal Life Force Energy in full body sessions on a regular basis, profound changes are bound to happen. In all likelihood you will become what you essentially always are: a free, sane and healthy individual, and not be conned any more (if you ever were) to remain the passive and uninformed consumer who takes everything at face value and refrains from challenging anyone who has ursurped the authority that is actually yours. Quite the contrary, you will take matters regarding your health in your own hands, and your life will become much the better for it.

Such profound changes usually don't occur overnight. They unfold gradually, and Reiki will remain your dependable companion until they are complete.

O'Brien,
Oregon,
July 23 1998

SUGGESTED READING

Arnold, Larry, and Sany Nevius. *Reiki Handbook: A Manual For Students And Therapists Of The Usui Ryoho System Of Healing.* PSI Press, 1982

Baginski, Bodo and Shalila Sharamon. *Reiki: Universal Life Energy.* Mendocino: LifeRhythm, 1988

Barnett, Libby and Maggie Chambers. *Reiki Energy Medicine: Bringing The Healing Touch Into Home, Hospital, and Hospice.* Rochester, Vermont, Healing Arts Press, 1996

Eos, Nancy, M.D. *Reiki And Medicine.* Grass Lake, Michigan: Eos, 1995

Gleisner, Earlene F. *Reiki In Everyday Living: How Universal Energy Is A Natural Part Of Life, Medicine, and Personal Growth.* Laytonville, California: White Feather Press, 1992

Haberly, Helen. *Reiki: Hawayo Takata's Story.* Olney, Maryland: Archedigm Publications, 1990

Horan, Paula. *Empowerment Through Reiki: The Path To Personal And Global Transformation.* Wilmot, Wisconsin, Lotus Light,1990

Horan, Paula. *Abundance Through Reiki.* Twin Lakes, Wisconsin: Lotus Light, 1995

Narrin, Janeanne. *One Degree Beyond: A Reiki Journey Into Energy Medicine.* Seattle, Washington: Little White Buffalo Publishing Cottage, 1997

All of my teaching is about helping people wake up. Students often ask me about my favorite books to help them go deeper in their own process. The following is an informal reading list taken from my book *Core Empowerment: A Course In The Power Of The Heart, With Commentaries For Advanced Reiki Practitioners*, which is a good introduction to my work with prospective Reiki masters and people who are seeking true Freedom, true Self.

For those who want to delve into the real roots of Reiki and learn more about the *Tantra Of The Lightening Flash Which Heals The Body And Illumines The Mind* from which Reiki is derived, the upcoming books by Lama Drugpa Yeshe Thrinley Odzer are highly recommended. Much of the translated material from Dr. Usui's own journals will also be included. My forthcoming book *True Reiki True Self* will include my own introduction to this body of knowledge.

All of Shri H.W.L. Poonja's (better known as Papaji) books come highly recommended: Every morning I start my day with reading a paragraph from *The Truth Is* which contains Satsang dialogues which cut right to the core between Papaji and his students. They are not only powerful evocations of non-duality, they are also filled with divine Love and Grace. *Papaji Interviews*, edited by David Godman, features longer interviews with western therapists. *Wake Up And Roar I* and *Wake Up And Roar II* contain further material from Papaji's Satsangs in Lucknow. These books are indeed precious because they are the voice of direct experience. Soon Papaji's biography in three volumes will be released under the title *Nothing Ever Happened*.

Whatever was collected of Ramana Maharshi's spoken words from many different authors is worth your time. Ramana was one of the greatest Realizer's of Supreme Reality in our time. He is also my own master's master, and T.S. Anantha Murthy wrote a beautiful biography of this sage's life called *The Life and Teachings of Sri Ramana Maharshi*. Another jewel in the literature of applied non-duality are Nisargadatta's books *I Am That* and *The Ultimate Medicine*. I can also recommend any of the books available with the dialogues of Ramesh Balsakar, who like Papaji and his teacher Nisargadatta were influenced by Ramana Maharshi. All of these teachers focus on vichar (direct self inquiry) which is the supreme yoga

The Benedictine monk Bede Griffiths, a one time student of C.S. Lewis, lived in India for many years in his ashram Shantivanam in Tamil Nadu and wrote many beautiful books about ultimate reality, taking into account a Christian perspective. I especially love *Return To The Center*, *A New Vision Of Reality*, and *Universal Wisdom*.

From the many Tibetan works on non-duality, either from a Sutra or Tantra approach available in English language I specifically wish to recommend Nyoshul Khenpo's *Great Perfection* and Namkhai Norbu's *The Crystal And The Way Of Light*. Many more titles are available, and if you are interested browse in a specialty bookstore in books presenting the teachings of Dzogchen and Mahamudra.

Finally, to get into the mood and get a first glimpse of what non-duality might entail, I can recommend all books of Wayne Dyer and Stuart Wilde. They are fun to read, very instructive and ideal particularly for the western reader (or the eastern reader with a western education and lifestyle) who has little background in applied non-duality and what it might mean, but plenty of curiosity and a true beginner's spirit, in the Zen sense that we all are always beginners because every moment is a new moment.

PAULA'S REIKI LINEAGE

Dr. Mikao Usui
Dr. Chujiro Hayashi
Hawayo Takata
Barbara Weber Ray
Maureen O'Toole
(who was trained by Mrs. Takata and Barbara Ray)
Kate Nani

ABOUT THE AUTHOR

Paula Horan is a psychologist, Reiki Master, author and seminar leader whose warmth and inspirational teaching help motivate her students to manifest the richness inherent in their lives. Over the past several years she has spent much time with her master Shri H.W.L. Poonjaji in India, a self realized being. Inspired by Him, she shifted her focus from self improvement to self inquiry.

At this point, her greatest gift to her students and readers is her ability to share the Freedom of true Self which is common to us all in every moment of our seemingly separate lives. She teaches *Reiki,* the *Core Abundance Seminar* and the *Core Empowerment Training* in several different countries, although she also enjoys the peace and quiet of a semi-secluded lifestyle.

Born in America, she lived her childhood years in Italy and Germany. She completed her undergraduate studies with a B.A. in sociology and English literature in Britain, and then passed both her M.A. (focusing on dance therapy) and her Ph.D. in psychology in San Diego, California.

Paula has appeared on Radio and T.V. shows in the U.S., Europe and India. Her first book, *Empowerment Through Reiki* has been translated into fifteen languages. It was followed by *Abundance Through Reiki* which was released in 1995. Recently, she released her third book *Core Empowerment: A Course In The Power Of The Heart,* which is actually a thorough revision and expansion of an earlier work, previously published under the title of *Dissolving Co-Dependency.*

Reiki— 108 Questions And Answers, Your Dependable Guide For A Lifetime Of Reiki Practice is her fourth book on a subject that continues to inspire so many people all around the globe.

In 1998, Paula was initiated into the *Men Chhos Rei Kei* master level by Lama Drugpa Yeshe Thrinley Odzer. *Men Chhos Rei Kei* is a complete system of advanced healing practices based on the *Tantra Of The Lightening Flash That Heals The Body And Illumines The Mind* and Dr. Usui's own teachings as transmitted by himself and his foremost student, Dr. Watanabe Yoshi.

Paula welcomes the questions and feedback of her readers. She answers every letter personally, although it may take a few months for the answer to reach its destination due to her frequent travels. Please, send all inquiries regarding this book, or requests for seminar schedules in India, or your interest in organizing a seminar to:

Reiki — 108 Questions And Answers
c/o FULL CIRCLE BOOKSHOP
34, Santushti Complex
New Delhi 110003
Tel.: (011) 688-1304 or 688-1306; Fax 688-1301

> **To be informed about Paula Horan's periodic visits to India contact:**
> Mumbai: (022) 617-4851; Delhi: (011) 686-2807

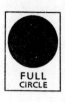

FULL CIRCLE

CORE EMPOWERMENT
A Course In The Power Of Heart
With Commentaries For
Advanced REIKI Practitioners
PAULA HORAN

The intention of this book is to inspire and help the reader appreciate whatever is happening in the moment, as the infinite play of Universal Life Force Energy. The motivation is not exactly to make the reader feel happy or good in the normal sense, but to experience what can only be described as non-causal joy; much like a sure faith and confidence that all is well, regardless of the way things may appear. In actual fact, feeling good or happy can easily turn out to be one of the many benefits of *Core Empowerment*.

As you read this book, you will notice that each chapter has a complementary essay regarding Reiki, the theme of which is always a spin- off on the intention of the accompanying chapter. Each chapter also has an exercise section which directly bears on the discussion in the text. These exercises are not meant to propel you into any kind of altered state, or new or better reality than the one you are experiencing now. The intention of these exercises is simply to help you fine tune your power.

ISBN 81-7621-029-3

FULL CIRCLE

The Curative Powers of the Holy Gita

T.R. Seshadri

...When disappointment stares me in the face and all alone I see not one ray of light, I go back to the Bhagvad-Gita. I find a verse here and a verse there, and immediately begin to smile in the midst of overwhelming tragedies — and my life has been full of external tragedies — and if they have left no visible, no indelible scar on me, I owe it all to the teaching of the Bhagavad-Gita...

— **Mahatma Gandhi**

No evil, however great, can affect him who meditates on the Gita. He is like the lotus leaf untouched by the water.

— **Varaha Purana**

Happiness is not possible without good health and good health is a state of mind. Dr. Seshadri offers a well-structured and easily comprehensible formula for good health using the Gita as the tenet for his theory. **In this book are given select verses which have the power to heal almost any disease if recited with complete faith.** You have to surrender in "total faith" and recite the verses to attain a state of good health. This is not a therapy but a process of "faith healing". It is not a substitute but a supplement to all regular medical therapies "Believe and you will achieve," says Dr. Seshadri and this book articulates the role of faith and mind-power in curing pathological manifestations which we know as diseases.

ISBN 81-216-0697-7